THE JUDGE'S GAVEL

Winning the Drug War by Empowering Recovery

- *New Terms of Engagement* -

Judith Ann Miller, Ph.D.
&
Diana Eccher, M.A.

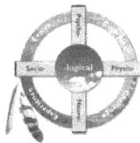

Soaring Hope Recovery
Colorado Springs, CO

ISBN: 978-0-578-58558-1

Library of Congress Control Number: 2020903297

This book is not intended to diagnose any medical conditions or to replace a healthcare professional.

Printed in the United States of America.

First printing edition 2020.

Soaring Hope Recovery
41250 Alford Road
Simla, CO 80835

SoaringHopeRecovery.com

For everyone that has endured incarceration because they suffer the disease of addiction.

CONTENTS

PREFACE

Addiction is not a crime!

We the people have the power, the science, and the technology to implement successful New Terms of Engagement for the War on Drugs. We desperately need new rules to dictate how we fight this devastating war, because the law of order for the past 50 years has only resulted in an extremely costly failure.

Presidents, legislators, and players of the judicial system must continue to fight the War on Drugs with a science-based plan of attack, and bestow the Judge's Gavel with the power of recovery — to win the war.

Addiction is a disease with an onset, a progression, and ends in death.

A Cunning Baffling Disease

Bill W. and Dr. Bob described alcoholism as cunning and baffling, in the Big Book. Perhaps the most important line in their book was: *More will be revealed*. Well, more has been revealed. Science has evolved to a neurological understanding of how alcoholism and drug addiction actually works and that it is indeed a brain disease.

> Addiction is a disease of the brain that affects the circuits involved in processing punishment and reward and in exerting inhibitory control. As a result, the addicted person will seek drugs compulsively even when they consciously don't want to and despite the threat of severe punishment, such as incarceration and loss of child custody, and at the expense of natural reinforcers, such as family and friends (Volkow, 2002). **Even despite the threat of death.**

The consequences are disturbing, and addiction is still in control.

> This malfunction in the brain enables addiction to prematurely end lives, ruin dreams, destroy families, and leave those suffering full of hopelessness, shame and guilt.

> Victims become lost and alone, disconnected from who they really are and who they dreamt they could be.

> If the pre-frontal cortex is impaired (dysfunctional), *the gate keeper of the brain* for decision making and strategic thinking, it cannot stop an urge or impulse from going straight to action.

> This is because the brain acts as a supercomputer that controls all of our thoughts, emotions, behaviors, and everyday actions. If it isn't functioning properly, addiction can be difficult to beat.

> (Whitney, 2020)

Addiction today has grown to epidemic (crisis) levels, has killed millions, continues to kill millions more, and leaves friends and family with forever heartaches. Our government created the failing War on Drugs, criminalized addiction, and it is now naively attempting to resolve the epidemic with new drugs... **Medication** Assisted Therapies (MAT).

Journalist Ajay Sinjh (2018) states that, "Addiction is destined to endure as one of the world's least understood and mistreated social maladies."

Today's addict faces a double jeopardy, created by the US Government:

1. Criminalization of their disease

2. Medicalized treatment that merely treats symptoms

Neither addresses the causes of addiction and therefore cannot be the answer to the epidemic. Incarceration and sanctions are not cures or viable solutions. Punishment and criminal treatment does not work, as the Department of Corrections is not designed to correct addiction.

New Terms of Engagement

New laws must redefine the roles of judicial players and how legislators can pass new *strategies* for engagement.

The President of the United States – Non-profit foundations fighting for reform and State level initiatives are proving that we the people do not have to sit around and wait (or hope) that out President will make the evidence-based changes that are needed to win this war. Former Presidents initiated and supported the War on Drugs, but we have the power to recognize past mistakes and pivot this war towards success, healing, and recovery.

National and State Legislators – It is imperative for senators and congress to fully understand addiction. They must realize that an addicted offender cannot willfully choose whether or not he/she drinks or uses drugs.

Modern and highly advanced brain function imaging visually proves that addiction is in fact a brain disease that hijacks a person's free will. We must focus on the neuroscientific evidence and Work With The Brain to Make The Changes, not chemically assault or traumatize it further.

An addicted person is like a person driving a vehicle without brakes:

The driver believes he is in control.
He can go fast or slow, or turn left or right with no problem...
But when he wants to stop – he can't because there are no brakes.

– Dr. Nora Volkow, NIDA Director, May 2009 –

Drug Court Judges – Our judges are bound by the legislative actions that created mandatory sentencing. It is encouraging that judges do have the power to sentence an addicted offender to treatment, rather than incarceration. However, this only applies to addicted offenders who have the financial means (about $100,000) to pay for a private attorney, allowable court costs, and then subsequently pays for their recovery treatment. A re-allocation of funds for incarceration over to treatment will allow judges to funnel addicts into recovery, regardless of income.

District Attorneys – DAs and ADAs are law keepers serving as crutches for a judge to determine sentencing. Addicted offenders are often threatened and mislead by mandatory detention laws, forcing them to accept an overwhelming, expensive, and expansive plea deal, regardless of guilt.

Defending Attorneys – A new set of rules will be invaluable for defending attorneys to represent their addicted clients. The rules and laws of the drug war that do not work bind today's defense attorneys. Public defenders are assigned too many cases at once, and they often funnel their clients through the path of least resistance… a complicated and expensive plea deal. The amount of clients/cases that a PD handles at any one time should be capped and limited, so they actually have time to represent each and every client to the best of their abilities.

Probation and Parole Officers – It is essential that criminal justice officers have science-based evaluation tools, training in evidence-based and dual-diagnosis addiction recovery methods, and a full understanding of how a sustainable treatment regime works. We also need stronger regulations for private probation and monitoring companies, to ensure they are not reaching outside evidence-based protocols, or abusing their government granted authoritative power.

Addiction Treatment Providers – Providing a sustainable SUD recovery treatment program requires a science-based model of care, and adequate consistent funding. Treatment for substance use disorders and co-morbid mental health issues will never be a one-size-fits-all protocol, because we are dealing with individual people with dizzying arrays of symptoms.

Medicalization (MAT) – Our medications have a rightful place in emergency, short-term, life-saving administration needs. However, to date there is no medication that is specifically designed to treat the causes of addiction. The pharmaceutical approach to addiction treatment merely treats addiction symptoms, and actually prolongs the disease causing serious and sometimes deadly side-effects. The perceived benefits of these prescriptions do not outweigh the harms.

The National Institute on Alcohol and Drug Abuse states that alcoholism and addiction entail severe imbalances in the neurotransmissions that create thought, and control behavior. An alcoholic/addict believes, with every cell in their body and every neuron in his brain, that his/her survival – literally, their survival – depends on use of alcohol or drugs.

In 2006, Nora Volkow, M.D., was called to testify before the U.S. House of Representatives Committee on the Judiciary. Dr. Volkow is a pioneer of photo-imaging technology, which allows us to see the actual workings of brains and the virtual creation of thought. Dr. Volkow is also the director of the aforementioned National Institute Of Drug Abuse in Washington, D.C. and was named Innovator of the Year in 2008. Her understanding of addiction is scientifically-based and is profound:

> The circuits involved in punishment and reward are circuits that are in our brain in order to motivate behaviors that are indispensable for survival. Drugs activate exactly the same circuits, but in much more efficient ways. When a person becomes addicted, those circuits signal to the brain the equivalent of: *you need to use the drug to survive*. The person that is addicted in that process seeks the drug not out of pleasure, but out of need.

> The value of punishment... when the signal is one of survival, becomes pale in comparison. An addicted person will seek his/her drug regardless of the catastrophic consequences. And that is a message extraordinarily important when the criminal justice system asks, "We cannot affect the behavior by punishment?"

> Well, the brain is not responding the same way it would, had that person not been affected by the drugs.

The Paradigm Shift – A proposal to eliminate the criminalization of the disease of addiction and shift treatment to non-pharmaceutical, science-based, evidence-based, value-based treatments. A tried and true model of care that works, providing sustainable recovery.

Chapter 1
Breaking The Chains

3 Hots and a Cot, plus Meds!

**Violence, Fear, Rape, Murder...

Incarceration Aftermath – The 3 Choices:

1. I've learned my lesson and will never use again

2. Re-offend (which most do)

3. Commit suicide (which many do)

There is no picture perfect moment when addiction sinks its barbed-wire claws in; it only etches out a disturbing footprint. Full-fledged addiction transpires much like the process of slow boiling a live turtle, death or wrongdoing is imminent, but it is not realized. It creeps in like a demon in the night and slowly takes control of the brain's ability to make choices.

People do not aspire to become addicts, and no one claims that the ride through the revolving criminal justice doors is amusing. In the song *Running to Stand Still* (1987) by rock band U2, the lyrics reverberate a poetic truth, that addiction is a constant fight against a force that physically pushes back. In desperate situations, people will intentionally break laws and self-incarcerate, simply to obtain a legal place to lie down and have food brought to their starving bellies. Either way, somewhere along the line, something went terribly wrong in their life, and alcohol, illicit drugs, and/or prescription medications were the only known, pushed, or available coping tools.

Most people naively continue their substance use with the belief that they are not addicted, or addiction will not happen to them. They will lean on drugs and alcohol until they find themselves in desperate situations, and eventually law enforcement yanks them out of the boiling water. Renowned psychiatrist, Dr. Nora Volkow of NIDA, points out that, "When drug abusers enter the criminal justice system, it signals a pivotal crisis in their lives, and it offers a unique opportunity to establish treatment for drug abuse and addiction."

The legal system can step in using punishment and fear to stop illicit behavior, for a short time, but the underlying issues causing addiction have already begun to fester; the proverbial demon is still attached and eager to wreak havoc. As of 2015, the largest private prison corporations, Core Civic and GEO Group, collectively manage over half of the private prison contracts in the United States with combined revenues of $3.5 billion (Gotsch & Basti, 2018). These contracts can easily be diverted to science-based residential recovery programs.

American singer-songwriter Johnny Cash gives a powerful review of the system's ability to reform inmates with his song *San Quentin* (1969). Cash explains that prison is a literal living hell, one that deteriorates the human spirit while educating the criminal mindset. What if an addict genuinely decides to live in recovery, and truly desires to do the work to become a healthy and productive member of society? The idea of prison was born in order to contain and monitor that small percentage of anti-social sociopaths, the deviant souls that intentionally harm others without any feelings of guilt or remorse. Some countries have even taken the initiative to begin studying, imaging, and possibly understanding the bizarre brains of these extreme societal outliers.

The United States holds nearly 25% of the global prison population (not including immigrant detainees), completely outpacing population growth and crime rates (World Population Review, 2019). This makes us a world champion in the practice of mass incarceration, but this is not a victory march. In July of 2019, Rep. Karen Bass stated, "It's really an embarrassment in our country that we have more people locked up in the United States than any place in the world."

Incarceration is a societal knee-jerk reaction to any wrong-doing, but the A&E television docuseries *60 Days In* (Henry, Woodard, & Grogan, 2016--) reveals that even a few hours as an inmate is in fact an overtly traumatic and terrifying experience for most people. The criminal justice system is successful in giving the aloof or entitled individual a reality check, and great at containing infamous and violent criminals that require maximum security, but it was not designed to house and rehabilitate mental illness and addiction. We simply cannot heal a broken mind by placing it in a fight, flight, or freeze mode, and then trap it in an uncaring, raucous, and demeaning environment with zero sense of safety. In this situation, the brain automatically reverts to survival mode, battle mode, and yes, addiction mode.

Public opinion has shifted dramatically in favor of sensible reforms that expand health-based approaches while reducing the role of criminalization in drug policy. As a nation, we are exhausted and fed up with the drug war's endless cycle of crime, community destruction, political corruption, mass incarceration, and legal discrimination.

Let's take a realistic look at the failure of the War on Drugs, the damage that the addicted offender suffers during incarceration, and the alarming yo-yo effect of criminal justice supervised intervention programs.

In 1951, President Truman signs The Boggs Act, stamping mandatory minimum sentencing into federal law. Pushing judicial discretion aside, a mandatory prison sentence for all drug related convictions became a requirement. Within two months, over 500 citizens were arrested under the provisions of the new law. A first-offense marijuana possession charge carried a minimum prison sentence of 2 to 10 years, with a fine of up to $20,000. Twenty years of arrests runs rampant, destroying families and communities, and President Nixon unwisely declares an official *War on Drugs*. The U.S. eventually imprisons the four main architects of Nixon's drug policy, because of the Watergate scandal. Is it irony that criminals conceived the War on Drugs?

In 1982, the Reagan administration ushered in a new Executive Order for the War on Drugs. The New Order made radical changes to drug policy and cut funding for addiction treatment programs. In turn, the demand for illicit drugs reaches insatiable levels, the world's most notorious and violent drug lords plant roots, and citizens become collateral damage. The nation experienced record numbers of drug overdoses, and the number of people behind bars for nonviolent drug offenses increased from 50,000 in 1980 to over 400,000 by 1997 (Drug Policy Alliance, 2020).

President Reagan permanently altered drug policy and persuaded politics, the courts, law enforcement, and American culture to blindly accept zero tolerance ideologies and drug-free fantasies. Nancy's "Just Say No" anti-drug campaign effectively spread ignorance and fear across the nation, teaching youth that drugs will either make you fly or they will fry your brain like an egg. If only we could go back in time and teach her that a developing or suppressed prefrontal cortex has limited control over a 'just say no' decision.

During the George W. Bush era, the nation witnessed a rapid escalation of the militarization of domestic drug law enforcement. By the end of his presidential term, Americans had endured tens of thousands of paramilitary-style SWAT raids, mostly for nonviolent drug offenses, which were often petty misdemeanor charges. Although the beginning of state-level reforms finally initiated a small reprieve, slowing the growth of the drug war. Many states are following suit today, by downgrading minor crimes and pushing for decriminalization across the nation.

Politicians now openly admit to past recreational drug use, as President Obama candidly said, "When I was a kid, I inhaled frequently – that was the point." During Michael Bloomberg's 2001 mayoral campaign he admits, "You bet I did – and I enjoyed it." Yet the assault on American citizens and others continues. The Trump administration is literally building a border wall, on the assumption that a physical barrier will keep drugs and crime out of the country. President Trump demanded harsher sentences for drug law violations and believes that a death penalty for people who sell drugs would stop trafficking. Yet he also rallied the public to resurrect the disproven "just say no" strategy to combat the opioid crisis.

We have the power to build a future where science and compassion shaped drug policy, rather than allowing political hysteria to decide our fate.

A great-suggested read is a book titled *The New Jim Crow: Mass Incarceration in the Age of Colorblindness* (2010), by Michelle Alexander, a civil rights litigator and legal scholar. Alexander shows that, by targeting black men through the War on Drugs and decimating communities of color, the U.S. criminal justice system functions as a contemporary system of racial control. It is perfectly legal to discriminate against convicted criminals in nearly all the ways in which it was once legal to discriminate against African Americans. Once labeled a felon, even for a minor drug crime, the old forms of discrimination are suddenly legal again. In her words, "we have not ended racial caste in America; we have merely redesigned it."

Another thought provoking read is a book titled *Chasing the Scream: The First and Last Days of the War on Drugs* (2015), by Johann Hari. The writing enlightens readers by detailing the ramifications of the drug war. For example, Hari illustrates how the Mafia created an extensive drug market that became the swindle of the century. "The lawmakers must have known that their edict, if enforced, was the clear equivalent of an order to create an illicit drug industry. They must have known that they were in effect ordering a company of drug smugglers into existence."

Johann Hari's book also eloquently presents the damage and devastation endured by victims of the war on drugs. He tells the heart-wrenching account of Billie Holiday's life of drugs, and the gut-wrenching story of Tent City in the deadly heat of Arizona, which ends in harsh criminal punishments. The book is a chapter after chapter absolute page-turner on the criminalization of addiction, and it will definitely cause tears to trickle down your face.

The 50-year war on drugs has cost the United States an estimated $1 trillion. In 2015, the federal government spent an estimated $9.2 million every day to incarcerate people charged with drug-related offenses, which is more than $3.3 billion per year (US Department of Justice, 2016). State governments spent another $7 billion in 2015 to incarcerate individuals for drug-related charges (Henderson & Delaney, 2017). Decades long tough on crime tradition forcefully demonized, criminalized, and imprisoned anyone that falls victim to a substance use disorder, and unilaterally uplifted drug dealing as a dangerous but extremely tempting career path. Marijuana legalization alone would save roughly $7.7 billion per year in averted enforcement costs, and would yield an additional $6 billion in tax revenue (Edwards & McCray, 2012). That $13.7 billion could place more than half a million people in evidence-based treatment programs, every year.

While the 13 years of the Volstead Act (1920-1933) did result in a number of positives, it is extremely difficult to recognize any positive results from the war on drugs. We cannot eliminate drug use and addiction by incarcerating everyone; we can't even keep drugs and alcohol out of our prisons. Slowly, and sometimes with great reluctance, judges today are opting to offer drug offenders a choice of treatment rather than incarceration, but incarceration with lighter sentencing is still the norm. Addiction is preventable and treatable, but the Science of Recovery is not practiced in jails and prisons, therefore, the Department of Corrections does not correct addiction. It is time to learn from our history of mistakes and join Johann Hari in the fight to, "End the war on drugs, and make sure people with addiction problems receive love and compassion instead of shame and stigma."

Dr. Nora Volkow is the director of the National Institute on Drug Abuse, which is part of the National Institutes of Health. Dr. Volkow pioneered the use of brain imaging to investigate the effects of drugs in the human brain, successfully demonstrating that drug addiction is a brain disease. More specifically, she reported that addiction is in fact a *disease of free will*, whereas drugs damage the brain's reward circuits, leaving people with dysfunctional brain pathways.

The following is an excerpt of her testimony (NIDA, 2019):

> I've thought about this many times, and I realize that describing addiction as a 'chronic brain disease' is a very theoretical and abstract concept. To explain the devastating changes in behavior of a person who is addicted, such that even the most severe threat of punishment is insufficient to keep them from taking drugs—where they are willing to give up *everything they care for* in order to take a drug—it is not enough to say that addiction is a chronic brain disease.

> What we mean by that is something very specific and profound: that because of drug use, a person's brain is no longer able to

produce something needed for functioning, and that healthy people take for granted, **free will**.

All drugs of abuse, whether legal or illegal, cause large surges of dopamine in brain areas crucial for motivating our behavior — both the reward regions as well as prefrontal regions that control our higher functions like judgment, decision making, and self-control over our actions. These brain circuits adapt to these surges by becoming much less sensitive to dopamine.

The result is that ordinary healthy things in our lives, all the pleasurable social and physical behaviors necessary for our survival (which are rewarded by small bursts of dopamine throughout the day) no longer are enough to motivate a person. The person needs the big surge of dopamine from the drug just to feel temporarily okay, and they must continually repeat this, in an endless vicious cycle.

We can do much to reduce the shame and the stigma of drug addiction, once medical professionals, and we as a society, understand that addiction is not just a disease of the brain, but one in which the circuits that enable us to exert free will no longer function as they should. Drugs disrupt these circuits. The person who is addicted does not choose to be addicted; it is no longer a choice to take the drug.

Once people understand the underlying pathology of addiction, people with the disease will not have to go through obstacles to obtain evidence-based treatments but will simply, non-judgmentally, receive the help they need, like a child with diabetes or a person with heart disease or cancer. They won't have to feel that shame, or feel inferior, because people understand that they are suffering from a disease that should be treated like any other.

Everyone suffering from a disease deserves treatment, but even with decades of overwhelming scientific proof, addiction is still believed to be simply a moral weakness deserving of grave punishment. "It is important to distinguish the fact that the addict does what he or she does, **not** to wreck their lives or the lives of others. Addictive behaviors are used as a means to cope with something that is simply not working right – that always ends up wrongly" (Stratton, 2019).

When people are sick, isolated, and miserable, they often turn to drugs to alter a disturbed state of mind, unknowingly handing over their own free will. It makes sense that pushing more pain, shame, and isolation onto an addict only worsens things, hurling him or her further into addiction.

Judith Miller, PhD, describes a conversation that she witnessed at one of her residential rehab facilities:

> Whilst making my daily rounds, I walked into the kitchen to see one of our new female clients sitting on the floor, wrapped up in a blanket with her back against the oven door. She looked up at me and cried out, "I have never felt so much pain in my life!"

> A young male client decided to join us, and took a seat beside her on the floor. He looked at her and explained, "You are so fortunate to be in a nice warm house, wrapped in a snuggly blanket, and surrounded by people who care. I detoxed from heroin, naked in a cold jail cell, with no blanket because I was suicidal. I had so much pain that I actually bit the bars. I am so glad to be here and have a comfortable clean bed without a stinky pillow, good nutritious food, and I don't ever have to eat a green bologna sandwich again."

> Another female client who was looking on chimed in, "I agree with everything he said, but the best part for me is that there is nobody masturbating at my bedside."

> I reached my hand down to the blanketed woman and said, "You're safe here, let me help you."

It is recognized that addiction is a brain disease, which is treatable and preventable, so perhaps reallocating funds from correctional institutions to science-based treatment programs is a logical step forward. While addicts are still being sentenced to imprisonment today, there is great hope for tomorrow. Author and journalist Johann Hari remarks that, "When the government war on alcohol stopped, the gangster war for alcohol stopped."

In 2006, The National Institute on Drug Abuse (NIDA) and the National Institutes of Health (NIH) released a landmark scientific report showing that effective treatment of drug abuse and addiction can save communities money and reduce crime. Here is an excerpt:

> It is estimated that 70% of individuals in state prisons and local jails have abused drugs regularly, compared to approximately 9% of the general population. Studies show that treatment cuts drug abuse in half, reduces criminal activity up to 80%, and reduces arrests up to 64%. However, less than one-fifth of these offenders receive treatment.

> Treatment not only lowers recidivism rates, it is also cost effective. It is estimated that for every dollar spent on addiction treatment programs, there is a $4 to $7 reduction in the cost of drug-related crimes. With some outpatient programs, total savings can exceed costs by a ratio of 12:1. The failure to treat addicts in the criminal justice system contributes to a continuous cycle of substance abuse and crime.

> "Detox alone in jail or prison is not treatment," said Dr. Nora Volkow. Without proven treatment and therapeutic follow-up in a community setting, addicted offenders are at a high risk of relapse despite a long period of forced sobriety. These principles also apply to court-mandated treatment interventions that replace incarceration with community programs.

> Access the full report on the NIH government website.

The outrageous and unwarranted costs required for contacting family while incarcerated, to make bail, or to participate in a release-treatment program are all predatory cash collecting avenues. Many jails actually implement a booking fee and a bond fee, so people are paying fees to be arrested and then paying fees in order to pay their release bond. Sound a bit excessive? These are just more consequences that broken people and their families endure because we allow our justice system to treat crime and punishment as a financially incentivized business.

Contrary to those who believe that privatized supervision and probation are too lenient in punishment, only a small percentage of offenders are currently placed in these alternative release-treatment programs.

At judgment day, if a person is lucky enough to qualify for 'alternative' sentencing or privatized supervision, they often end up feeling betrayed and develop immense regret for even wanting recovery. The alternative sentencing 'treatment' programs are designed as another disciplinary arm of the criminal justice business. These programs are an overwhelming extension of the court's punitive powers, along with supervising officers who still function under the premise of catching criminals.

It is a myth that empowering and expanding parole, probation, pretrial, and privatized supervision will reduce incarceration populations. Alternative punishments might look lenient on paper, but in practice, they have proven to be gateway sentences. Granted most people would prefer to remain in the community instead of sitting in jail, but these programs set people up to fail. Many people find themselves not being able to afford the costs, or incurring violations due to minor infractions.

In 2016, the Prison Policy Initiative reported:

> At least 168,000 people were incarcerated for such "technical violations" of probation or parole — that is, not for any new crime. It is important to minimize the punitive power of court mandated programs, reforming them with resources to support and reward success. Having supervision in place to simply detect

mistakes only leads to unnecessary time in confinement, which in turn threatens any forward movement achieved from working a treatment program.

Addiction is a vicious cycle in itself, and incarceration or court supervised treatment programs for addicts and the mentally ill have only intensified the complexity of this problem. We need to unravel the strings of mental dysfunction, not tie increasingly complex knots in it. If addiction thrives in negativity, then requiring an addict to endure the stigma of criminal supervision and believing that their addiction can heal with a dark cloud of incarceration always on the horizon is foolish.

The past several decades have witnessed an increased interest in providing substance abuse treatment services, but only a small percentage of offenders have access to adequate services, especially in jails and community correctional facilities (Taxman et al., 2007 & Sabol et al., 2010). Not only is there a gap in the availability of these services for offenders, but also there are often few choices in the types of services provided. Treatment that is of insufficient quality and intensity, or that is not well suited to the needs of offenders may not yield meaningful reductions in drug use and recidivism.

Untreated offenders are more likely to relapse to drug abuse and return to criminal behavior. This can lead to re-arrest and re-incarceration, while jeopardizing public health and public safety, and taxing criminal justice system resources.

We must empower the American Justice System to relinquish control of the rehabilitation aspect, and allow judges to place people in science-based, dual-diagnosis facilities.

A rehab facility done correctly has the same initial outcome as incarceration in the way that we are pulling addicted offenders out of society. The difference is that these broken people will have access to private therapists, healing resources based in science, and a safe environment conducive to a sustainable recovery.

In a Studio10 interview (2015), Johann Hari explains:

> The opposite of addiction is not sobriety; the opposite of addiction is connection. Human beings have an innate need to bond and connect, and when we are happy and healthy we'll bond and connect with each other. Addiction is about not being able to bear being present in your life.

The reason some people do not use drugs is not because anyone is stopping them, they do not use because those people *want* to be present in their lives. They have work that is meaningful to them, people they love, connections they care about, and things in life that *need* them to be present.

In our science-based recovery program, our first priority with clients is to help them change their attitudes. Many arrive with the perception that they are victims, not of a disease, but of law enforcement.

We provide specific education and counseling to cultivate an understanding of the harm done to their families, their communities, and themselves. Given that level of understanding, we can support our clients through the legal process and work with attorneys, district attorneys, law enforcement, parole officers, probation officers, and public defenders... to ensure that people have a chance to negotiate a path of justice as part of their recovery. They can return to society, not with a criminal or victim mindset, but with a positive and hopeful view of the future. The case for treating drug and alcohol abusing offenders is compelling.

As the timeless Bob Marley preached inner peace and serenity to the masses, it is time to give people with addiction and mental health issues the chance to write their own *Redemption Song* (1980).

THE RAT PARK EXPERIMENTS
(ALEXANDER, 1981)

What Does "Rat Park" Teach Us About Addiction?

We owe to American psychologist, Dr Bruce Alexander, the understanding that addiction is about far more than any drug. That a person (or animal) in his studies is an active ingredient in their interaction with any drug. To stand a chance beating the opioid and other drug epidemics we have, we will be far better equipped if we follow his lead.

Alexander's experiments, in the 1970s, have come to be called the "Rat Park." Researchers had already proved that when rats were placed in a cage, all alone, with no other community of rats, and offered two water bottles—one filled with water and the other with heroin or cocaine—the rats would repetitively drink from the drug-laced bottles until they all overdosed and died. Like pigeons pressing a pleasure lever, they were relentless, until their bodies and brains were overcome, and they died.

But Alexander wondered: is this about the drug or might it be related to the setting they were in? To test his hypothesis, he put rats in "rat parks," where they were among others and free to roam and play, to socialize and to have sex. And they were given the same access to the same two types of drug-laced bottles. When inhabiting a "rat park," they remarkably preferred the plain water. Even when they did imbibe from the drug-filled bottle, they did so intermittently, not obsessively, and never overdosed. **A social community beat the power of drugs.**

(Sederer, 2019).

Dr. Sederer is an Adjunct Professor of Epidemiology at Columbia University Mailman School of Public Health, a distinguished Psychiatrist Advisor to the New York State Office of Mental Health (OMH), and the Director of Columbia Psychiatry Media.

Chapter 2
Decriminalize Mental Disorders

Insanity: mental illness of a severe nature when a person cannot distinguish fantasy from reality, cannot conduct her/his affairs due to psychosis, or is subject to **uncontrollable impulsive behavior.**

A cocktail of medications only alters the communication network and delicate chemical balance of a highly complex behavioral system that we do not fully understand.

The phrase "tough on crime" is a common platitude used by politicians in order to gain donations, votes, and support from the public. In order to make society safer and more secure, we need to address why uncontrollable criminal behavior is happening, and then provide non-pharmaceutical evidence-based treatment to people *before* their issues turn catastrophic.

"When we think of addicts, we very seldom associate them with the word discrimination. Scientific research has proven that addiction is a chronic medical condition and not an issue of moral integrity, but there remains a global perspective that an addict is morally weak or compromised" (Brown, 2019).

Addiction is a disease that leads to criminal behavior, although addiction is not the root of the problem. The real issue begins with the underlying causes, as people are generally drawn to alcohol, drugs, and risky behavior because of their biological, psychological, and environmental conditions.

It should be recognized that these underlying causes are not crimes to be punished; they are neurological dysfunctions that require specific, dual-diagnosis, science-based treatment programs.

One of the nation's leading neuroscience and addiction journalists, Maia Szalavitz writes, "The number one cause of addiction stigma is the fact that drugs are criminalized. We don't lock people up with diabetes when they eat a donut, or lock depressed people up when they are sad, therefore, we cannot criminalize people for having an addiction" (Szalavitz, 2016).

Maia suggests:

- Decriminalize the possession of substances.

- Expunge drug war related criminal records.

- Use the money spent to criminalize drug offenders to pay for evidence-based treatment with experienced, evolved, compassionate and supporting therapists.

We must accept the fact that our jails, prisons, institutions, and criminal justice services are overflowing with individuals who have brains that are just not working well. A dysfunctional and/or damaged brain causes an impaired ability to participate in all the things that healthy people take for granted, such as therapy, morality, love, empathy, decision making, and even free will.

It is time to renew, reform, and ultimately decriminalize addiction and mental health disorders. The justice system is simply not designed to treat the brain. Too many offenders are suffering from varying degrees of physical brain injuries, traumatic stress, anxiety disorders, depression, and substance use disorders, which are often the underlying causes of criminal behavior.

Common Myths About Addiction

Myth: People with addiction are criminals and deserve punishment.

Myth: Addiction is a behavioral and moral problem, not a disease.

Myth: Shame and punishment is the only way to handle a relapse.

Myth: Prescription drugs are not dangerous if they come from a doctor.

Myth: Medication is necessary for addiction recovery.

Myth: Using drugs or alcohol is a choice, so addiction is their own fault.

Myth: If they just use willpower, they can stop using.

The following pages list common mental health conditions that are frequently self-medicated, or exacerbated by prescription medications, or both—all contributing to excessive substance use leading to destructive and criminal behaviors.

Adverse Childhood Experiences (ACE)

All types of abuse, neglect, and other traumatic experiences that happen to people under the age of 18, before the brain is fully developed, have substantial negative effects on learning, behavior, and physiology. The toxic stress from these experiences harms a child's developing brain and body so profoundly that they suffer repercussions long into adulthood.

Childhood trauma often manifests in adults as chronic disease, mental illness, learning disorders, behavioral issues, addiction, victimization, and violence. Children raised in or around substance abuse manufacture poor coping skills, existential fears, negative attitudes, family role confusion, and are eight times more likely to succumb to a chemical addiction themselves.

A vulnerable and unprotected growing mind becomes maladaptive if it is not protected from adult situations and problems. Experiences from the past shape future behavior.

Adverse childhood experiences include:

- In utero trauma
- Abandonment
- Emotionally absent parent
- No rules, boundaries, or limitations
- Government Detention
- Head Injury
- Emotional abuse
- Physical abuse
- Sexual abuse
- Emotional neglect
- Physical neglect

- Bullying (on and off-line)
- Exposure to violence
- Abuse of mother or sibling
- Household substance abuse
- Household mental illness
- Incarcerated household member
- Continual police presence
- Parental death, separation, or divorce
- Family member attempt or commit suicide

Such experiences change how a child's brain responds to stress, and they internalize them as reference points. Repeated intense experiences, such as violence and abuse, eventually numb or dull a child's healthy emotional reactions to these situations.

Any adverse childhood experience puts people at a much higher risk for negative mental and physical health conditions, and life outcomes as adults (Hampton, 2019). Many children tend to find comfort from unmanaged stress through excessive eating, violent video games, unruly behavior, and emotional detachment.

Prenatal Risk Factors – Heavy alcohol exposure to a fetus physically damages the brain cells, which alters a child's behavioral development.

Any toxin introduced to an unborn baby carries a high risk for damage to healthy cells, be it consumed by the mother, or induced by her body. Excessive testosterone exposure in the womb can create a predisposition to violence and aggression, often leading to abnormally high levels of the hormone into adulthood.

Attention Deficit Disorder (ADD/ADHD)

A neurological developmental disorder that can be a barrier to academic and career success. People with ADHD generally experience difficulty staying focused and paying attention, difficulty controlling behavior, and hyperactivity (SAMHSA, 2019). It is expected that both genetic factors as well as environmental influences play a role in the development of ADHD (Soreff, 2019).

Primary symptoms include: a constant need for physical activity, inattentiveness, and impulsivity.

> **Symptoms related to inattention**: trouble paying attention in school or work, the appearance of not listening, avoidance of activities that require sustained focus, losing things, and being easily distracted.

> **Symptoms related to hyperactivity**: restlessness, fidgeting, interrupting, frequent talking, intrusiveness, trouble paying attention, and trying to do multiple things at once.

Other symptoms include: insomnia, low tolerance to frustration, poor self-image, forgetfulness, disorganization, and mood swings. Hyper-focus can also be a symptom, which is a tendency to intensely focus on one task or event that precludes focus on necessary tasks.

Psychostimulant medications are often prescribed for ADHD. Dr. Anne Procyk (2018) reports a significant number of ADHD cases are simply the result of blood sugar swings, and regulating blood sugar can cure an affected person. She first suggests a healthy, balanced diet. Also, determining if there is an essential fatty acid and magnesium deficiency, getting adequate amounts of refreshing sleep, and daily strenuous exercise is essential. Dr. Procyk warns that stimulant medications can further diminish hunger signals and exacerbate blood sugar swings, which results in worsening symptoms, leading to higher medication doses, thus contributing to a vicious cycle.

Post-Traumatic Stress (PTSD)

PTSD is one of the most diagnosed disorders in the world, as people are often exposed to extreme trauma that is difficult to heal. Traumatic stress develops after witnessing or experiencing a very stressful, frightening, or distressing event, or after a prolonged traumatic experience, and it is the lingering effect of such trauma that turns into a stress disorder.

Examples include:

- Physical or sexual assault
- Prolonged physical, mental, or emotional abuse
- War and conflict
- Incarceration, captivity, or torture
- Burglary or home invasion
- Natural disasters
- Serious accidents and injuries
- Being in a life-threatening situation
- Serious health problems
- Childbirth experiences, such as losing a baby
- Exposure to traumatic work events, including remotely
- Homelessness or starvation

Post-Traumatic Stress **symptoms** are easily recognized as: sleeplessness, irrational anger, suicidal ideation, flashbacks, hyper-vigilance, nightmares, difficulty concentrating or focusing, dissociation from reality, panic attacks (Corry, 2008).

The judicial system must face the realization that all veterans suffer varying degrees of PTSD, caused by military experiences, which becomes the underlying cause of addiction, leading to criminal behavior.

Non-military persons also suffer PTSD, caused by any traumatic experience. Any person, of any age, or gender can develop this stress disorder he or she experiences or witnesses a traumatic or violent event.

About one half of all U.S. adults experience at least one traumatic event in their lifetime, but many do not develop a disorder. PTSD is not usually related to situations that are simply upsetting, such as divorce, job loss or failing exams.

People who experience Post-Traumatic Stress may have persistent, frightening thoughts and memories of the event(s), experience sleep problems, feel detached or numb, or may be easily startled. In severe forms, PTSD can significantly impair the ability to function at work, home, and socially (SAMHSA, 2019).

Working or living in an outdated, mismanaged, or poorly regulated jail or prison puts officers, staff, visitors, and inmates in danger of developing this stress disorder.

Laura Greenstein (2017) of the
National Alliance in Mental Illness (NAMI) states:

> When we think about post-traumatic stress disorder, it's typically in the context of active duty service members and veterans—for good reason. Dangerous and potentially traumatic situations are common occurrences in the context of military service.
>
> However, it is important to note that PTSD is not exclusive to this type of trauma. In the U.S., about eight million people experience PTSD. If people believe that only service members and veterans can develop PTSD, the recognition of symptoms and treatment can be delayed.

Antidepressant, Antianxiety, and Antipsychotic medications are often prescribed in an educated guess, or on a trial and error basis to treat the symptoms caused by Traumatic Stress.

Traumatic Brain Injury (TBI)

Almost everyone has experienced a head injury or mild concussion, be it through a fall or smack to the head, just by living a normal life. A traumatic brain injury usually results from a violent blow or jolt to the head or body, or when an object pierces the skull and enters brain tissue.

These injuries often result in long-term complications, changes in mental state, and sometimes end in coma or death. Military personnel, athletes, construction workers, automobile accident victims, assault victims, and people not wearing helmets often acquire these extreme head injuries. In 2014, the Center for Disease Control reported 'falls' as the leading cause of traumatic brain injuries in the United States. Although, many head injuries that occur in professional sports go unreported.

Traumatic brain injuries often impact language and motor skills (Corry, 2008). TBI is associated with higher impulsivity, aggressive behavior, and negative emotions (Frost & Hedges, 2013).

If a TBI is suspected, **call 911 immediately** or take the person to an emergency room. TBI Disabilities generally include:

- Problems with cognition (thinking, memory, reasoning)
- Sensory processing (sight, hearing, touch, taste, smell)
- Communication (expression and understanding)
- Behavioral and mental health issues (depression, anxiety, personality changes, aggression, acting out, and socially inappropriate behavior)
- Migraines or headaches

The Brain Injury Alliance of Colorado (BIAC) envisions a place in which all survivors can thrive, including those that have been or are currently involved in the criminal justice system. Research shows that incarcerated individuals are seven times more likely to have experienced a brain injury than the general population. The goal is to offer support for these individuals, so they may improve their quality of life and strengthen the greater community.

Incarcerated individuals with brain injuries have:

- Greater risk of mental health disorders
- More likely to abuse substances
- Greater risk of suicidal ideation & attempts
- 50% higher rate of recidivism
- Lower treatment completion rates
- Higher rates of disciplinary incidents

The following is the **slew of medications** often used to alter/treat the symptoms of a traumatic brain injury:

Analgesics (**Opioids**): for pain relief and pain management.
Antianxiety (**Benzos, SSRIs**): for uncertainty, nervousness, fear.
Anticoagulants (Blood Thinners): to prevent blood clots.
Anticonvulsants (**Barbs, Benzos, Opioids**): to prevent seizures.
Antidepressants (**SSRIs**): for depression and anxiety.
Antipsychotics (**Tranquilizers**): for combativeness & hallucinations.
Muscle Relaxants (**Benzos**): to reduce muscle spasms or spasticity.
Sedative-Hypnotics (**Benzos, Z-drugs**): to induce sleep.
Stimulants (**Amphetamines**): to increase alertness and attention.

Chronic Traumatic Encephalopathy (CTE) is a neurodegenerative disease caused by repeated head injuries, which are commonly observed in contact sports such as football, hockey, and boxing. Symptoms include behavioral problems, mood problems, problems thinking overall, psychosis, and suicide. Symptoms typically do not begin until years after the injuries. CTE often gets worse over time and can result in dementia.

Generalized Anxiety Disorder (GAD)

GAD is the most common type of all anxiety (or stress) disorders. It is characterized by excessive and persistent worry and tension, even without an identifiable cause. The intensity of this type of anxiety can interfere with all aspects of a person's life, and impair their ability to function optimally on a daily basis.

The usual course of GAD is chronic with symptoms developing more slowly than other anxiety disorders, and females are twice as likely to be affected. The exact cause of this mental illness is unknown, but there is evidence that biological factors, family background, and life experiences, particularly stressful ones, play a role. When the anxiety is severe, some people can have difficulty carrying out the simplest daily activities. Many believe that worry prevents bad things from happening, so they view it as risky to give up their worry. Some people even struggle with physical symptoms such as stomachaches and headaches from their constant stress and worry.

An anxiety attack is an intense and/or extended period of anxiety. It is more severe than the simple feeling of anxiety, but less severe than a panic attack. It can last anywhere from minutes to hours, even days and weeks. The Diagnostic and Statistical Manual of Mental Disorders (DSM-5) defines a panic attack as, "A sudden episode of intense fear that triggers severe physical reactions when there is no real danger or apparent cause."

While everyone experiences stress to some degree, people with an anxiety disorder become obsessed with feelings or thoughts that they cannot control. Medications are widely prescribed to those suffering anxiety, and in many cases, the **side effects** of these drugs contribute to increased anxiety and depression. The underlying causes of anxiety must be considered in order to provide relief. Research has shown that the major causes of anxiety are magnesium deficiency, adrenal dysfunction, inadequate sleep, hormonal imbalance, and hypoglycemia (Procyk, 2018).

In May 2019, the American Psychiatric Association reported that for the second year in a row, two out of three Americans say they are "extremely or somewhat anxious" about their health, paying bills, and keeping themselves and their family safe.

Neuroscientist Joseph LeDoux believes that a true understanding of anxiety lies in an exploration of one of the most complex subjects left in neuroscience: The nature of consciousness (the subject of his recent book, *The Deep History of Ourselves: The Four-Billion-Year Story of How We Got Conscious Brains*, 2019).

The brain's amygdala primes the body to react defensively by activating hormonal cascades and defensive behaviors. The mind, or higher-level processing parts of the brain is where we form our beliefs and give meaning to what we experience. In a way, the emotions that we call "fear" and "anxiety" are manifestations of our consciousness. Any truly effective treatment for anxiety, LeDoux (2019) argues, will require a better understanding of processes beyond the ancient brain structures that trigger behaviors and release hormones, extending to what creates our awareness of self.

The last big anti-anxiety medication was Prozac and other selective serotonin reuptake inhibitors, or SSRIs, which came out in the 1980s. The awkward truth about current anxiety treatments is that they are for the most part unproven. Benzodiazepines suppress activity in the fear centers of the brain by downregulating key neurotransmitters, but also suppress them everywhere else. They cause sedation, locomotor movement suppression, respiratory suppression, and cognitive impairments, among other things.

Kay Tye, neuroscientist at Salk Institute for Biological Sciences (2019) states: "We're just bathing the brain and body in these drugs. And, when you take a drug systemically, it's going to go through your circulatory system. It's going to pass through the blood brain barrier. And it's going to bathe the entire tangled mess of wires that is our brain in a soup."

Major Depressive Disorder (Clinical Depression)

One in five (about 46.6 million) Americans live with a mental illness, and depression is the most commonly diagnosed behavioral health issue. Depression is also the most complicated of all emotions, and yet the most common psychological problem one can experience.

It is a persistent feeling of gloom or sadness that is usually accompanied by a slowing down of the body. When a depressed mood becomes so severe that it interferes with normal daily activities that are necessary to maintain interpersonal relationships, work or daily life, it is identified as a mental disorder.

Symptoms of major depression (Harvard Health, 2018) include:

- Distinctly depressed or irritable mood
- Loss of interest or pleasure
- Decreased or increased weight or appetite
- Decreased or increased sleep
- Appearing slowed or agitated
- Fatigue and loss of energy
- Feeling worthless or guilty
- Poor concentration or indecisiveness
- Thoughts of death, suicide attempts or plans

Depression may present in one of four patterns:

- Substance Induced Depression caused by the use, abuse, and addiction to alcohol and drugs (legal or illegal).
- Depression Induced Substance Abuse occurs when people suffering from depressive illness self-medicate with alcohol or drugs to manage their symptoms and become dependent upon those substances.

- Situational Depression occurs when a person experiences a traumatic event, or extreme stress.

- Co-occurring Depressive Illness occurs when a person suffers from substance use disorder and an independent depressive illness. The depression is temporarily relieved during drinking or drugging, but then returns to a severe form when seeking sobriety.

Research has shown that low serotonin is the major cause of depression.

Antidepressant medication is often prescribed for depression, but only on a trial and error basis because each individual system reacts differently to these chemicals. Dr. Anne Procyk asserts, "The key to understanding someone's depression is understanding why the serotonin is low, not just giving an SSRI to make the serotonin last longer."

Dr. Procyk acknowledges that Prozac may help, but identifying why it is needed is key to figuring out a real cure. It is essential to cure the problem rather than manage the problem.

Issues to consider are (Procyk, 2018):

- B-vitamin insufficiency

- Adequate protein

- Long-term use of acid-blocking medications

- Thyroid functioning

- Optimal vitamin D

- Adequate exercise

- Fatty acid deficiency

- Adequate amounts of refreshing sleep

*Seasonal Affective Disorder (SAD) is a type of depression associated with the changes in seasons, especially experienced during the winter months. This disorder zaps energy and creates moodiness. Better known as the winter blues, it can cause increased anxiety, sadness and stress, lack of enjoyment in regular activities, feelings of isolation, mood swings, and several other symptoms that can take over one's life. SAD affects over 10 million people in the U.S. (Boston University, 2019).

Insomnia

A sleep disorder (inability to experience restful sleep) often caused by stress, anxiety, medications, caffeine, and certain medical conditions. Dr. Katherine George (2019) reports the potential causes of insomnia:

- **Anxiety** – The Mayo Clinic notes that trouble sleeping is one of the most common symptoms of an anxiety disorder. This condition can greatly affect sleeping by causing a racing heartbeat and/or night terrors.

  "Additionally, there are people who experience what are called nocturnal panic attacks, meaning they may have transient episodes of intense panic that wake them up from their slumber," says Dr. Okeke-Igbokwe.

- **Alcohol** – Some believe alcohol helps them sleep, but it actually has the opposite effect. Alcohol causes people to wake up more easily in the second half of their sleep. It is also more likely to wake you up to use the bathroom, which interrupts sleep.

- **Vitamin D Deficiency** – Someone who lacks the proper amount of vitamin D, may be losing sleep. This can lead to a slew of health problems including cardiovascular disease, cancer, weak bones, and poor sleep.

- **Sleep Apnea** – A common culprit behind the lack of sleep. This condition causes people to wake up, or experience shallow breathing throughout the night.

- **Overactive Thyroid** – This butterfly shaped gland located in the front of the neck is responsible for almost all of the metabolic processes in the body.

  An overactive thyroid could be to blame for sleep troubles.

- **Age** – There are many things that change with age, and sleep is one of them. Older people find that when they start getting into bed earlier, they fall asleep easily.

- **Excess Belly Fat** – Living with excess stomach fat can create all kinds of problems for someone's health, including their ability to sleep soundly.

- **Nocturia** – There is nothing worse than waking up from a wonderful deep sleep because of a full bladder.

- **Eating Before Bed** – Eating too close to bedtime can make it difficult to fall asleep or stay asleep.

Sleep deprivation makes it difficult for brain cells to communicate effectively, which in turn, can lead to temporary mental lapses that affect memory, judgment, and visual perception.

Insomnia causes people to take **stimulant** drugs to stay alert during the day, **sedative** drugs to wind down, and **Z-drugs** to artificially induce sleep during the night. In the short term, a lack of adequate sleep can affect judgment, mood, ability to learn and retain information, and may increase the risk of serious accidents and injury. In the long term, chronic sleep deprivation may lead to a host of health problems including obesity, diabetes, cardiovascular disease, and even early mortality.

Bipolar Disorder (Manic Depression)

Bipolar disorder is a serious brain disorder that causes unusual shifts in mood, energy, activity levels, thought processing speed, and the ability to carry out day-to-day tasks. People with Bipolar I or II experience phases of mania or hypomania, and major depressive episodes.

People with bipolar disorder may misuse alcohol or drugs, have relationship problems, or perform poorly in school or at work. Family, friends, and people experiencing symptoms may not recognize these problems as signs of a major mental illness such as bipolar disorder (National Institute of Mental Health, 2016).

Mania & Hypomania:

- Grandiose delusions
- Highly confident
- Decreased sleep needs
- Trouble sleeping
- Boundless energy
- Restless mind
- Over-talkative
- Flight of ideas
- Distractibility
- Goal-directed behavior
- Risky behavior
- Feeling immortal

Depression:

- Introverted
- Negative attitude
- Problems concentrating
- Lack of energy
- Thinking slows
- Negative focus on past
- Anxiety or panic
- Loss of confidence
- Low self-esteem
- Oversleeping & tiredness
- Loss of interest
- Full-body muscle tightness

Depressive symptoms are present nearly every day for a period of two weeks, sometimes much longer. The lows of bipolar depression are often so debilitating that people may be unable to get out of bed. When people are depressed to this extreme, even a minor a decision such as what to eat for a meal is overwhelming. During a depressive episode, people become obsessed with feelings of loss, personal failure, guilt or helplessness. It is important to note that this cycle of negative thinking can lead to thoughts of suicide.

A manic episode lasts for about a week, and hypomanic episodes last for about four days. Mania symptoms are more severe, showing obvious impairment with possible psychosis or even hospitalization.

Research links higher levels of aggression and anger attacks, with a Bipolar Disorder. Violent behaviors in bipolar individuals generally only occur co-morbidly with a substance use disorder, or during a rare psychotic episode. The dramatic shifts in mood, energy, and activity levels associated with Bipolar Disorder are more severe than the normal ups and downs experienced by everyone.

Medications for Bipolar are generally a lifelong regiment of multiple:

- Anticonvulsants (**Barbiturates**, **Benzodiazepines**, **Opioids**)
- Antipsychotics (**Tranquilizers**)
- Antidepressants (**SSRIs**)
- Anti-anxiety (**Benzos, SSRIs**)

Medications are generally prescribed on a trial and error basis.

Bipolar symptoms appear when brain chemistry is severely disrupted. Many of these issues can be relieved with a healthy, nutritious diet. If the only treatment given is increased or new medications, this will not fix the problem and symptoms will continue to escalate (Procyk, 2018).

Social Anxiety Disorder (Social Phobia)

Social anxiety is often confused with shyness, but this disorder is actually an intense fear of social situations, which ultimately involves interaction with other people. It is a deeply rooted fear of being watched and negatively judged by other people.

The main difference between social and avoidance disorders is that people with social anxiety disorder usually know that their fears are irrational.

A person with an avoidance personality disorder believes that s/he is inferior to others, making rejection and humiliation not only inevitable, but also deserved.

In a group setting, or being watched by others, phobias tend to manifest (National Institute of Mental Health, 2016) as:

- Blushing, sweating, shaking, pounding heart, mind going blank.

- Experiencing vertigo, feeling nauseous or faint.

- Tight and rigid body posture, making little eye contact, and speaking with a quaking or overly soft voice.

- Finding it scary and difficult to be with other people, especially those they do not already know, and have a hard time talking to them even though they wish they could.

- Being very self-conscious in front of other people and feeling embarrassed and awkward.

- Being very afraid that other people will judge them.

- Staying away from places where there are other people.

Underdeveloped social skills are a possible contributor to social anxiety, since misunderstanding the behavior of others may play a role in causing or worsening symptoms, but several parts of the brain are involved in fear and anxiety.

Many doctors recommend beta-blockers or benzodiazepine prescriptions to provide temporary relief from anxiety and social phobias, but this does not solve the problem. Social fears only occur in certain situations, so prescribing addictive drugs or long-term antidepressants for these intermittent occurrences is obviously more harmful than beneficial. Scientists can create better treatments with funding and better resources to explore exactly how fear and anxiety work in the brain.

About 20% of people with social anxiety disorder also suffer from alcohol abuse or dependence, and a recent study found that the two disorders have a stronger connection among women (ADAA).

Dr. Murray Stein and John Walker, PhD, write in *Triumph Over Shyness: Conquering Social Anxiety Disorder* (2009) that social anxiety disorder "frequently travels in the company of other emotional difficulties," such as alcohol or drug abuse, depression, and other anxiety disorders.

Although alcohol can temporarily reduce symptoms of social anxiety – which is the reason many turn to it – Stein and Walker note that alcohol can also increase anxiety, irritability, or depression a few hours later or the next day. Even moderate amounts of alcohol can affect one's mood and anxiety level.

*Antisocial Personality Disorder (ASPD)** is a mental condition in which a person has a long-term pattern of manipulating, exploiting, or violating the rights of others without any remorse (DSM-5). Those with ASPD often acquire biological anomalies in their brain, which in turn impairs their moral conscience.

Many people use the expression "anti-social" to describe an introvert or a person who does not enjoy group activities. Unsocial or asocial are better terms to describe a shy, socially awkward, or non-talkative personality.

Asperger Syndrome (AD)

Asperger's is a rare condition that is sometimes viewed as a hidden disorder. Depending on the severity of symptoms, affected individuals may either exhibit unusual social behavior, or be severely impaired in their social and professional life.

Despite normal and sometimes superior intelligence, people with Asperger's have difficulty understanding social conventions and reading social cues. As a result, they often seem insensitive or rude, and making friends can be hard for them. No two people experience this disorder in the same way.

Social Interaction – People with this condition tend to find social situations very confusing, and many times do not have the ability to understand social cues. They have difficulty deciding things such as whose turn it is to talk next, when to finish talking, how long to talk for, how long to maintain eye contact, and what the boundaries are in a conversation. They tend to simply avoid any type of social situation.

Social Thinking – Sometimes it is a struggle for them to figure out what another person is thinking, or gauge how they are feeling, although extreme emotions are quite clear.

Difficulty with Small Talk – Starting or engaging in meaningless conversations with strangers, or random people they encounter feels like a foreign concept.

Unintentional Rudeness – There is usually a great misunderstanding of social conversational boundaries, and Asperger's people sometimes lack tactfulness in a conversation causing them to say the wrong thing at the wrong time.

Difficulty Visualizing – It is generally a struggle to visually imagine spoken or written word details. Following oral directions can be frustrating and confusing.

Great with Fine Details – People with Asperger's are usually exceptional at noticing obscure details and minor changes, and remembering facts that interest them.

Obsessive Interests – Most people with this syndrome have very narrow and specific interests, causing them to over-indulge and learn everything about that one topic. Someone with Asperger's may utilize this symptom as a way to relax.

Hyper-focus – This is generally an obsessive or unusual ability to focus. To an observer it may appear as if the person is 'zoning-out' of reality or even lost, but they are actually internalizing and focusing-in, in great detail on something.

Need for Routine – This may be expressed as a need for a physical daily routine, a need to plan out activities, struggling with unanticipated change, or even simply a need to complete a task in a specific way.

Less common issues are Palilalia (repeating or 'mouthing' spoken words), physical ticks, both obsessive and compulsive, taking things literally, poor motor skills, overly sensitive to touch, and savant-like talents.

Asperger's is sometimes explained as a highly-functioning person on the varying degrees of the autism spectrum.

*Autism Spectrum is considered a developmental disorder that affects communication and behavior. Autism can be diagnosed at any age, but it is a "developmental" disorder because symptoms generally appear in the first two years of life. Autism refers to a broad range of conditions that are characterized by challenges with social skills, repetitive behaviors, speech and nonverbal communication. The ability to use language to express one's needs, and the ability to engage in social interaction is either nonexistent or highly underdeveloped.

Obsessive Compulsive Disorder (OCD)

OCD is identified as uncontrollable reoccurring thoughts (obsessions), and behaviors (compulsions) to repeat over and over (SAMHSA, 2019). Obsessive Compulsive Disorder may manifest in extreme behavior that is impossible to control with medication.

OCD requires complex thinking with a high I.Q., and results in seemingly absurd behavior such as counting steps, or breaths, or impulsive fixations on patterns, and may even create a feeling of wanting to die. Many sufferers believe that something catastrophic will happen if they do not complete an obsessive-compulsive task.

Research has found that serotonin as an anti-rumination chemical can cancel obsessive-compulsive behavior, and provide relief from this reoccurring affliction. It is noted that adequate amounts of serotonin are not provided by antidepressants. Holistic methods are more effective for providing relief from this disorder.

*Nomophobia is a term describing a growing fear in today's world—the fear of being without a mobile device, or beyond mobile phone contact.

*Agoraphobia – It is estimated that 5 to 20 million Americans suffer the symptoms, such as being afraid of life, and having lost the ability to control their perception of extreme sensory stimulus of their personal environment. They tend to stay indoors, avoid public places, and experience an over production of adrenaline. Medical treatment has traditionally been benzodiazepines to numb the unwanted feelings of dread and overpowering fear, and to slow the heart rate and respiration. Holistic treatment involves dietary modification to control the production of adrenaline, and slow stretching exercises to remove lactic acid.

Borderline Personality Disorder (BPD)

This is a mental illness characterized by a distorted self-image, impulsiveness, unstable and intense relationships, and extreme emotions. It presents as an enduring pattern of inner experience and behavior, which deviates markedly from the expectations of the individual's culture (SAMHSA, 2019).

Typically, signs of borderline personality disorder have developed by early adulthood, which is when most people experience the worst effects, and the condition may improve over time. This mental disorder is considered very common, with more than 3 million cases per year in the United States alone.

A common trait of individuals with personality disorders is unpredictable behavior, with no constant or typical reaction. They are more likely to make impulsive decisions and may be prone to odd habits such as walking in a specific direction or eating food in a specific order. A deviation from their set patterns can elicit a strong, negative reaction (Neil, 2019).

People with BPD find it challenging to regulate their emotions, which can result in self-harm behaviors. In addition, they may experience inappropriate, intense anger and mood swings that can last from a few hours to a few days. They also generally have a fear of abandonment, and will go to extreme measures to prevent real or imagined abandonment. This can lead to unstable and intense relationships, idolizing someone one minute, then thinking he or she does not care the next.

A feeling of emptiness is another characteristic of BPD. Individuals may lose contact with reality, engage in self-harming behaviors, threaten or attempt to take their own life, and engage in risky behaviors. General uncertainty and indecision can result in frequent changes to jobs, friends, goals, and values (Neil, 2019).

Premenstrual Dysphoric Disorder (PMDD)

Premenstrual syndrome (PMS) is a hormone-related health issue, **not a mental health disorder**, but we mention it because any type of chaotic hormone production does affect the brain, emotions, behavior, and overall health. This includes altering hormones with synthetics, contraceptives, medications, or drugs and alcohol.

PMDD is a more serious hormonal health problem that is similar to PMS. It causes extreme mood shifts and severe pain that can disrupt work, overwhelm everyday life, and damage relationships. It is heartbreaking and ultimately traumatizing for friends, family, and partners to witness their loved one experience these issues, and not be able to help. Unbalanced hormone production also causes irregular menstrual cycles, making symptoms very tough to recognize, predict, or treat at onset.

PMDD includes looping symptoms of extreme sadness, hopelessness, irritability, stress, anger, anxiety, intense abdominal cramping, irregular bleeding, headaches, and suicidal feelings, along with other common PMS symptoms such as breast tenderness and bloating.

There is very little medical research into this very real women's health issue, so trial and error hormonal treatments, dangerous and highly interactive contraceptive drugs, and mind-altering antidepressant chemicals are commonly prescribed to combat the debilitating symptoms.

Many women today are taking a noble leap and making the important decision to stop allowing these chemical assaults on their delicate systems. They are rightfully educating themselves about nutrition, overall women's health, and finding other successful treatment options, such as multi-nutrient treatments.

Members of The Alliance for Addiction Solutions (AFAS) have clinically observed that more women relapse premenstrually than they do at any other time of the month. We should not be surprised by this, as research data indicates that most arrested women tend to start their periods within a week of being put in jail (i.e. they commit their crimes during PMS).

Overall, this health issue is caused by an imbalance of estrogen and progesterone, as both drop towards baseline at the end of the cycle. There is a drop in serotonin levels as estrogen drops and a corresponding dysregulation in blood sugar levels.

Symptoms of low serotonin and rapidly dropping blood sugar levels include sugar cravings, tearfulness, irritability, rage, anxiety, agitation, obsessive thinking, fatigue, and insomnia. When blood sugar levels drop rapidly, there is a corresponding release of adrenaline (activation of the sympathetic nervous system) which reduces access to impulse control and the recovery skills stored in the prefrontal cortex.

Research has also shown that willpower drops as glucose levels drop in the prefrontal cortex. So, just at the same time as upsetting feelings increase, the ability to slow down, think through things, and access stress management skills decreases. Women are therefore at a very high risk to turn to the addictive behaviors which they familiarly and historically used to cope with stress.

Christina Veselak, LMFT, CN (2020), recommends avoiding refined sugars and starches, restoring blood sugar levels with The Pro-Recovery Diet, and the use of the amino acid l-glutamine. Recovering female addicts need to track their periods, eat extra protein during that time, get extra support, and increase their use of a serotonin precursor such as 5HTP if indicated. Many chronically relapsing women have found that these simple tactics completely eliminate their relapsing behaviors.

In a recent PhD study, conducted at the University of Canterbury, Christchurch clinical psychologist Dr. Hāna Retallick–Brown (2020) found that nutrients offer a viable, safe treatment option for women suffering from PMS. Her study revealed that using a single nutrient (vitamin B6), or even a micronutrient formula of blended vitamins and minerals achieved beneficial results, many participants experienced full remission from PMS symptoms.

Alcohol Use Disorder (Alcoholism)

A chronic and lifelong disease characterized by the inability to control drinking, stemming from physical and emotional dependence on alcohol.

This disorder causes people to experience a physically powerful need to drink, to continue drinking even under the threat of extreme consequences, and to suffer a rapid onset of dangerous withdrawal symptoms. These symptoms include headache, confusion, dizziness, irritability, racing heart, extreme anxiety, nightmares, and insomnia. Heavier drinkers may experience tremors (shakes), hallucinations, seizures, and delirium tremens (DTs).

Alcohol cravings are triggered by the exposure to any person, place, thing, or memory associated with drinking, but the most common physiological cause of an alcohol craving is hypoglycemia (low blood-sugar). Instead of the brain sending a healthy hunger signal, it essentially delivers an intense signal to drink.

The anxiety alcoholic differs from the hypoglycemic alcoholic in that anxiety is constantly present. This type of alcoholic may have been poisoned by excitotoxins, such as pesticides or heavy metals that continue to stimulate the nervous system. Many excitotoxins also lurk in most packaged, processed, and fast foods.

A second contributor to alcoholism is a genetic predisposition known as allergic-addicted, where a person lacks the enzyme to detoxify or metabolize alcohol. This allergic reaction causes the release of endorphins.

Another genetic contributor causes the body to convert alcohol to THIQ, which is a powerful opiate compound that is highly addictive. This is often seen in the person who can drink others under the table, and appears to be high rather than drunk.

Women tend to progress into alcoholism more rapidly because they absorb and metabolize alcohol differently from men. In the stomach, females simply produce less of the alcohol-metabolizing enzyme ADH (alcohol dehydrogenase), causing a larger proportion of ingested alcohol to reach the bloodstream. Women also retain a smaller amount of body water, so imagine the different concentration levels when dropping the same amount of alcohol into a smaller cup of water.

Given that fat does not directly absorb alcohol, women maintain higher concentrations of alcohol in their bloodstream, since they generally have a higher proportion of body fat than men do. Together with estrogen, these factors have a net concentrating effect on the alcohol in the blood, giving women a more intense hit with each drink. Therefore, women will have a higher blood alcohol content and experience greater intoxication than men per amount of alcohol consumed.

"This intense intoxication is so enjoyable that many (women) try to duplicate the experience over and over" (Lemonick, 2019).

Women and people with a lower body weight also have a greater risk of experiencing a blackout, even with lower levels of consumption. A blackout occurrence is fairly common for alcoholics that consistently drink to excess, binge drinkers, and for anyone that consumes alcohol too fast or drinks too much on an empty stomach. Consuming large amounts of alcohol to prepare for a drinking event is also a common way to induce a blackout occurrence.

Researchers have identified two unique types of blackouts:

En bloc, or complete blackout: This occurs when a drinker has an inability to recall entire events that occurred during the drinking session. En bloc blackouts happen when information is not successfully transferred from short-term to long-term memory during a drinking episode.

The person who is drinking can sufficiently keep information in short-term memory to engage in conversations, drive a car, and participate in other complicated activities. However, all this information is completely lost as the brain fails to transfer the person's short-term memory information to their long-term memory storage.

"The defining characteristic of a complete blackout is that memory loss is permanent and cannot be recalled under any circumstances" (Hildago, 2017).

Fragmentary-memory loss: This occurs when a drinker can only recall some portion of the events that occurred during the drinking session. Fragmentary blackouts are more common and occur when long-term memory formation is partially blocked.

Unlike en bloc blackouts, fragmentary blackouts allow for recall of all memories that were stored during the drinking event, but successful recall may involve a bit of effort and prompting.

What causes a blackout? Early studies on blackouts demonstrated that although alcohol is necessary for initiating a blackout, a large quantity of alcohol alone is not always the cause of a blackout. In fact, people sometimes have a blackout experience even when not drinking at their highest level.

Factors such as how alcohol is ingested, gender, and genetic susceptibility all play a role in determining a person's propensity for blackouts.

Head injuries, which many drinkers of all consumption levels tend to encounter during drinking sessions, can also cause memory loss.

Although, having a single blackout isn't always a sign or predictor of alcoholism, repeated blackouts are very often associated with having an alcohol use disorder, and being at risk for chronic alcoholism.

*Dissociative Identity Disorder (DID)** – Previously referred to as multiple personality disorder, this illness is usually a reaction to severe trauma as a way to help a person avoid or block terrible memories. Dissociative Identity Disorder is characterized by the presence of two or more distinct personality identities. Each persona may have a unique name, personal history, and characteristics.

Schizophrenia Spectrum Disorders

Persons experiencing schizophrenia suffer hallucinations, delusions, and unusual ways of thinking, as well as a reduced expression of emotions, reduced motivation to accomplish goals, difficulty in social relationships, motor impairment, and cognitive impairment (SAMHSA, 2019).

Schizophrenia and other psychotic disorders are of the most impairing forms of psychopathology, frequently associated with a profound negative effect on the individual's educational, occupational, and social function.

These disorders often manifest at the time of transition from adolescence to adulthood.

The spectrum of psychotic disorders includes (Barch & Ceaser, 2012):

- Schizophrenia
- Schizoaffective disorder
- Delusional disorder
- Schizotypal personality disorder
- Schizophreniform disorder
- Brief psychotic disorder
- Psychosis associated with substance or medical conditions

Substance-Induced Disorders

These disorders are peculiar because all or most of the psychiatric symptoms experienced are the direct result of substance use. The fact that the toxic effects of substances artificially create mental illness must be a revelation to the criminal justice system.

Simply put, substance use disorders and mental illness cannot be cured by shame or punished into remission and obedience.

The Diagnostic and Statistical Manual of Mental Disorders (DSM-5) lists the following:

- Substance-induced mood disorder
- Substance-induced anxiety disorder
- Substance-induced delirium
- Substance-induced persisting amnesia disorder
- Substance-induced sleep disorder
- Substance-induced persisting dementia
- Substance-induced psychotic disorder
- Hallucinogen persisting perceptual disorder
- Substance-induced sexual dysfunction

"Symptoms of substance-induced disorders run the gamut from mild anxiety and depression to full-blown manic and other psychotic reactions. Virtually any substance taken in very large quantities over a long enough period can lead to a psychotic state" (SAMHSA, 2005).

During a psychotic episode, an individual may experience hallucinations and/or delusions, and he/she usually isn't aware of his or her behavior. These episodes are quite common today with more than 200,000 U.S. cases per year.

Many substance-induced symptoms begin to improve within hours or days after substance use has stopped, but long-term effects and even permanent damage is possible. Some substances are directly toxic to the brain, such as alcohol, inhalants, and amphetamines.

Common classes of substances of abuse accompanying psychiatric symptoms seen in intoxication, withdrawal, or chronic use are:

- Alcohol
- Cocaine
- Amphetamines
- Hallucinogens
- Opioids
- Sedatives
- Caffeine
- Nicotine

"Some people who have what appear to be substance-induced disorders may turn out to have both a substance-induced disorder and an independent mental disorder. Assessment, treatment programs, and clinical staff can concentrate on screening for mental disorders, along with an understanding of the client's support network and overall life situation (SAMHSA, 2005).

Anyone with a presenting substance-induced disorder, be it from prescription medications, or legal drugs, or even illegal substance use, should be diverted to intensive medical treatment—before incarceration, and before criminal charges, judgement and sentencing is imposed.

Addiction is a complicated disease that affects the most complex organ in the human body, and people deserve proper assessment and treatment. When a person's mind is clear and functioning optimally again, then he/she can truly understand any wrongdoings and rightfully atone for them.

The Positive Social Impact of Decriminalizing Addiction

Substance abuse has a massive impact on serious social issues, which affects our everyday civilized society. Addiction is in our backyard, and the cowardly NIMBY tactic is for entitled people that fear the truth and deny scientific evidence. Do we continue to play this never-ending game of whac-a-mole, or can we adapt, evolve, and positively change the status quo?

PROTECTION & ENDING THE DISCRIMINATION

The American with Disabilities Act (ADA), the Rehabilitation Act, the Fair Housing Act (FHA), and other laws have been designed to protect against discrimination. While it is illegal under federal, state, and city law to discriminate against someone with a substance use disorder; the discrimination against individuals with addictions continues. Unlike someone with an obvious physical disability, those who suffer from substance abuse are less likely to garnish sympathy or receive compassion. They are more likely to receive unfair treatment from employers, the judicial and legal system, as well as the therapeutic and social service communities. It is illegal for an employer or anyone else to discriminate against an individual who is currently receiving treatment or has received treatment for addiction. Yet, discrimination does and continues to occur, and it is not always through blatant acts.

Have you ever watched the horror film *Saw* (Hoffman, Koules, & Burg, 2004)? It is understandable if you have not because there are some things in life that you just cannot un-see. The movie is obviously fiction, but if you think about the story with a critical mind, it actually reveals a grotesque mirror reflecting how people erroneously see addiction. The goal of the perverse *Saw* puzzles was to force addicts and criminals to "appreciate life" by facing death. If they figured out the puzzle and passed the test, survived, they were instantly cured of all their wicked behaviors and therefore worthy of their life and freedom. In reality, an addict's brain does not have the physical capacity to pass this test, but we continue to believe that our own undefeatable traps will somehow punish the wicked out of them.

People instinctively believe that an addict simply needs to change their thinking and appreciate the gift of life as everyone else does. However, once we label them as crazy addicts or scary criminals, their life will never be as everyone else's. Society will treat them like second-class citizens, void of any integrity or morality, and undeserving of basic human dignity.

We mentally torture addicts by incarcerating them, continue altering their brain chemistry with the latest and greatest medications, and then tie them down with lifelong records that report them as liars, liabilities, and villains. It really is not a wonder why drugs, alcohol, and addiction prevail because we rig the system to promote failure and hopelessness.

Our society utilizes criminal background checks before granting someone basic needs to operate in the world, and these investigative services only report the negatives. Maybe an addict seriously worked through an extensive but private treatment program, something the criminal justice system does not report? Moreover, because treatment is in fact a sensitive and private health issue, these positive efforts never reach consideration.

It is blatant discrimination for a business to deny an individual a non-driving job simply because their background check reports DUI charges on their record. One driving under the influence charge is likely a human error in judgment, but multiple charges are a failure on the system's end to recognize and offer sustainable treatment options for an obvious substance use disorder. We can apply this to any charge on a background check, because every situation has context, and most businesses use policy as an excuse not to investigate any positive aspects.

We flippantly criminalize addiction, and doom addicts to a lifetime of rejection. We ban them from any assistance, deny them affordable housing, limit occupational licensing, and handicap them in the employment race with a criminal record of bad behavior that is not always deliberate. All the while, we expect them to appreciate their life and freedom, respect and follow civility rules while enduring discrimination, and to function as regular productive 'members' of society.

Imagine for just a minute all of the possibilities for positive changes that could come from decriminalizing addiction. "Approximately 77 million Americans, or 1 in 3 adults, have a criminal record" (NCSL, 2018). If we just gift the survivors of this debilitating and deadly disease the chance to be functioning people again, most of these issues can change:

Shootings and Suicides – Every school and mass shooting over 2 decades, the shooters were on psychotropic medications, which incite aggression, violence, mood swings, hallucinations, confusion, suicidal thoughts, and more. The FDA utilizes a black-box warning on these prescription drugs because the evidence is overwhelming. Note that illicit and legal drugs also cause these brain dysfunctions.

Domestic Violence and Homicide – More than 3 women a day die by the hands of their own spouse. An average of 5 million acts of domestic violence occur annually to women aged 18 years and older, with over 3 million involving men. (Futures Without Violence, 2020).

Child Abuse and Neglect – The national rounded number of children who received a child protective services investigation response or alternative response increased 8.4% from 2014 (3,261,000) to 2018 (3,534,000). Stats do not include the many children that are not in the judicial system.

Divorce – For any marriage plagued with drug/alcohol abuse and excessive psychotropic medication divorce is eminent. One of our patients candidly reported, "I have had parties lasting longer than my 3 marriages."

DUIs/DWAIs – One of our patients had a brilliant epiphany, "It's funny, I haven't gotten a DUI since you helped me quit drinking!"

Drug Dealing & Theft – When an addict reaches the tipping point between hopelessness and rejection from the world, they relapse, period. They will steal and deal out of desperation to survive another day.

Bankruptcy and Homelessness – Could there be a correlation between substance abuse and bankruptcy stats? How many of our neighbors lose their home or employment due to incarceration, unwaivering probation or parole requirements, and criminal records? Hire a recovering addict on probation or parole, they will appreciate their job like none other.

Police Shootings – In the last 5 years, over 5,000 people died in a police shooting. How many police deaths occur because their job requires them to lock-up a desperate addict, instead of taking them to treatment?

Chapter 3
Drugs & Brain Dysfunction

Established about a century ago, the Brain-Dysfunction Theory continues to gain more evidence on a daily basis. This theory contends that illicit drugs, recreational drugs, and medication-assisted treatments disable normal brain function and actually cause generalized brain dysfunction.

Typical symptoms of substance-induced brain dysfunction, such as euphoria, apathy, and indifference are precursors to poor judgment and decision making, which leads to violence, suicide, and crime.

The most prevalent drugs and medications work to create neurological dysfunctions that lead to criminal behavior. Prescription medication changes the brain in lasting ways, and we must be conservative about using brain-altering drugs. Brain altering medications are generally not in the best interest of the person.

From the homely aspirin to the most sophisticated prescription medicine on the market, all drugs produce **side effects**. Many effects are minor, some are just an inconvenience, some are just plain strange, but many effects are very serious.

The Drug Enforcement Agency schedules drugs *because* they are known to be addictive with dangerous use outcomes:

Schedule I Drugs - Most dangerous, no medical use, high potential for abuse, leads to severe psychological or physical dependence.

Schedule II Drugs - Dangerous, high potential for abuse. Use potentially leads to severe psychological or physical dependence.

Schedule III Drugs - Potential for dependence.

Schedule IV Drugs - Risk of dependence.

Schedule V Drugs - Potential for abuse.

Part One: Recreational Drugs

All drugs have side-effects...
Addiction is about the brain, not the drug itself.

Sugar

Type: Stimulant
FDA Approved Legal Drug
Ingested

Sugar stimulates and depletes neurotransmitters in the brain similarly to cocaine, heroin, and ecstasy. The 'quick fix' sugar approach often leads to dramatic mood swings, and these unpredictable moods and behaviors are literally crazy making.

A diet filled with too many added sweeteners such as white sugar, honey, maple syrup, high-fructose corn syrup and molasses has a detrimental impact on physical and mental health.

Sugar affects learning and memory. After six weeks of drinking a fructose solution, much like soda, rats 'forgot' how to find their way out of a maze. Insulin resistance from a diet high in sugar damages the communication between brain cells responsible for learning and memory formation.

The rapid fluctuation of blood sugar often exacerbates mood disorder symptoms. High sugar intake leads to an increased risk of depression and can even worsen schizophrenia. Sugar may not increase the risk of anxiety, but it does worsen the symptoms, and deteriorates the mind and body, ultimately disrupting a person's ability to cope with stress.

Sugar's addictive potential has a growing amount of evidence. Drugs and sugar both flood the brain with a swift dopamine 'feel-good' kick. Research shows that rats prefer sugar-water over cocaine, and they also display classic signs of addiction without their sugary products, including tolerance and withdrawal.

The human mind and body were never designed to process immense amounts of sugar. Coping with addiction and mental disorders is already tricky without adding the sugar component.

Alcohol

Type: CNS Depressant (Sedative)
Legal Recreational Drug
Ingested or Absorbed

Consumable alcohol is often used to cover up and relieve emotional trauma and stress. Heavy drinking slowly leads to a life of chaos, complete loss of control, and catastrophic life and death consequences. Alcohol affects the brain much like rapid antidepressants do, interfering with the brain's communication pathways. These disruptions change mood and behavior, and make it difficult to think clearly and move with coordination.

Labels: Domestic, Craft, or Imported – Beer, Wine, Spirits.

Acute Effects: slurred speech, lack of coordination, mood and behavior changes, depression, and euphoria.

Health Risks: amnesia, addiction, liver damage, brain damage, heart failure, diabetes, cancer and infections.

Withdrawal – When a person suddenly stops drinking after prolonged and heavy use the brain functions like a runaway train. Symptoms include headaches, nightmares, anxiety, depression, hopelessness, body aches, shakes, nausea, intense cravings, tremors, hallucinations, and seizures.

Delirium Tremens (DTs) occur in about one out of every 20 people and are the most dangerous form of alcohol withdrawal.

In delirium tremens, the brain is not able to smoothly readjust its chemistry after alcohol is stopped. This creates a state of temporary confusion and leads to dangerous changes in the way the brain regulates circulation and breathing. The body's vital signs such as heart rate or blood pressure can change dramatically or unpredictably, creating a risk of heart attack, stroke or death (Harvard Health, 2019).

Prison Wine (Pruno, Hooch)

Type: CNS Depressant (Sedative)
Homemade Alcohol (Illegal without a permit)
Ingested or Absorbed

The name Pruno is derived from a once popular ingredient, prunes. Jailhouse hooch is fermented fruit juice made from moldy bread, oranges, and lots of sugar, which is then kept warm in showers, hidden in toilets, and generally strained through a used sock. Along with alcoholic effects, pruno also produces mild hallucinogenic effects.

Inmates in many prisons have contracted botulism (a rare and potentially deadly disease) from brewing and drinking the notorious prison wine. Botulism attacks the body's nerves and can lead to paralysis and death. The inmates interviewed often believed that illness from pruno was caused by others making the pruno wrong or using either rotten or unripe ingredients.

Some of the **symptoms of botulism** are: double vision, blurred vision, drooping eyelids, slurred speech, difficulty swallowing, thick-feeling tongue, dry mouth, muscle weakness, difficulty breathing.

Moonshine is called rotgut for a reason. Consuming too much alcohol can cause alcohol poisoning, affecting heart rate and breathing. Improperly distilled or adulterated Moonshine contains methyl alcohol, which is **highly toxic**. Direct ingestion of just 10mL can cause permanent brain damage and blindness by destruction of the optic nerve, and 30mL poisons the central nervous system leading to coma and probable death.

Names: Hooch, Juice, Brew, Raisin Jack, Chalk, Moonshine, Buck, Jump.

Someone who has suffered from alcohol use disorder in the past could be signing their death certificate drinking homemade booze. Steer clear of inexperienced distillers, untrustorthy people, and unsanitary conditions. It could be the difference between life and death.

Cigarettes & Tobacco

(Nicotine)
Type: Stimulant
Legal Drugs
Smoked, Vaporized, or Chewed (Absorbed)

Nicotine reaches the brain within 8 seconds of inhalation, affecting the neurotransmitter acetylcholine and its receptor. This receptor carries messages related to respiration, heart rate, memory, alertness, and muscle movement. These alterations in the brain cause a nicotine user to feel abnormal when not using, and to feel normal the user has to keep his or her body supplied with nicotine.

Nicotine activates the reward circuits in the brain, releasing a surge of dopamine and producing a pleasurable feeling, making a user crave this pleasurable behavior.

It also causes a decrease in the enzyme that is responsible for breaking down dopamine. The decrease in this enzyme results in higher-than-normal dopamine levels. These teeter-totter effects on dopamine push smokers to learn a powerful association with the good feelings from smoking—not only with cigarettes themselves, but also with things that remind them of smoking.

According to the National Institute on Drug Abuse, nicotine is a highly addictive substance, but it is actually the tobacco in nicotine products that can cause deadly cancers.

Acute Effects: increased heart rate and blood pressure, increased alertness, stress relief, a sense of well-being, and reduced appetite.

Withdrawal - Very intense cravings for nicotine, with tingling in the hands and feet, sweating, nausea and abdominal cramping, constipation and gas, headaches, coughing, sore throat, insomnia, difficulty concentrating, anxiety, irritability, depression, and weight gain.

THC (Marijuana)

(Tetrahydrocannabinol)
Type: Stimulant, Depressant, and Hallucinogen
DEA Schedule I Drug - Legal in some States
Smoked, Vaporized, Absorbed, or Ingested

THC is the addictive and principal psychoactive agent in cannabis, which is responsible for most of the plant's psychological effects. Many people use this drug to ease withdrawal symptoms, or as an alternative to other drug addictions. THC can over-activate the neural communication system, and heavy or chronic use often leads to impaired coordination and issues with problem solving, thinking, learning, and memory. For adolescents and young adults, the size and shape of the two brain regions involved in emotion and motivation are negatively impacted, even with experimental or recreational use. Heavy use at a young age alters brain development, and creates an increasing risk of developing mental health disorders, such as anxiety, depression, bipolar, or schizophrenia.

Labels: Indica, Sativa, or Hybrid - Flower, Concentrates, Oil, Liquid, Resin, Hash, Keif, Edibles, Topicals, Tinctures.

Acute Effects: euphoria, hyperfocus, relaxation, slowed reactions, altered perception, increased heart rate and appetite.

Health Risks: anxiety, panic attacks, delusions, chronic cough, frequent respiratory infections, and addiction.

Withdrawal - People suddenly stopping after heavy use tend to experience irritability, insomnia, and anxiety.

WARNING: Bootleg vape juice, e-liquid, and cartridges can contain Vitamin E acetate, or other oils, which will clog and shut down the lungs. Unregulated homegrown marijuana products can contain mold, mildew, mites, pesticides, and other dangerous additives.

**Pure CBD strains and Hemp do not produce psychoactive effects.

Kratom

(Mitragynine Extract)
Type: Stimulant and Depressant (Opioid)
DEA Unscheduled - Drug of Concern - FDA Warning
Ingested, Chewed, or Smoked

Kratom is a tropical tree with leaves containing compounds that induce mind-altering effects, and it is banned by some states in the U.S. due to safety concerns. The herb is currently easy to order on the Internet, and generally sold in packets labeled "not for human consumption." Two compounds in the leaves interact with opioid receptors in the brain, producing sedation, pleasure, and decreased pain, or stimulant effects depending on the dose. People use this drug recreationally, and some believe that it eases withdrawal symptoms and cravings caused by addiction to opioids, alcohol, or other substances. There is no scientific evidence that kratom is an effective or a safe alternative, it is in fact just as addictive and damaging as any other psychoactive drug.

Labels: Biak-Biak, Gratom, Ithang, Kakuam, Katawn, Kedemba, Ketum, Krathom, Kraton, Kratum, Maeng Da Leaf, Mambog, Thang.

Acute Effects: sedation, pleasure, and decreased pain (large dose); increased energy, sociability, and alertness (small dose).

Health Risks: tongue numbness, itching, sweating, nausea, vomiting, dry mouth, increased urination, constipation, aggression, seizures, hallucinations, delusions, psychosis, and thyroid problems. Kratom can worsen existing mental disorders, and users with these disorders appear to have an increased risk of suicide.

Withdrawal - As with any opiate-like drug, regular users experience decreased appetite, diarrhea, muscle pain, spasms, twitches, watery eyes, anxiety, anger, hot flashes, fever, insomnia, irritability, hostility, aggression, emotional changes, runny nose, and jerky movements.

Heroin

Type: Depressant (Opioid)
DEA Schedule I Drug
Injected, Snorted, or Smoked

Heroin is a cousin of both morphine and opium, and is chemically related to most prescription pain medications. Opiates enter the brain rapidly and bind to opioid receptors that are involved in feeling pain and pleasure, and those responsible for controlling heart rate, sleeping, and breathing. Opiates are highly addictive and regular users develop a tolerance, which means that they need higher and more frequent doses of the drug to satiate a craving. Users also tend to develop severe depression and personality disorders, along with the loss of brain white matter, which affects decision-making, behavior control, and responses to stressful situations.

Street names: H, Hero, Smack, Horse, Hell Dust, Brain Damage. Many slang terms are created based on the drug's appearance, packaging, effects, origin, or for deception.

Acute Effects: euphoria, dry mouth, severe itching, nausea and vomiting, analgesia, slowed breathing and heart rate, heavy feeling in the arms and legs, clouded mental functioning, in and out of consciousness.

Health Risks: addiction, insomnia, collapsed veins, abscesses, heart infection, constipation, stomach cramps, liver or kidney disease, pneumonia, and fatal overdose. There is always a risk of contracting HIV, hepatitis, and infectious diseases from using shared needles.

Withdrawal - Stopping this drug abruptly causes severe sickness, and can begin within just a few hours. People experience restlessness, severe muscle and bone pain, insomnia, diarrhea and vomiting, cold flashes, uncontrollable leg movements, and severe cravings.

Opium

Type: Depressant (Opioid)
DEA Schedule II Drug
Smoked, Injected, or Ingested

Opium is a narcotic depressant drug, which means it slows down the messages traveling between the brain and the body. Opiates are highly addictive and regular users develop a tolerance, which means that they need higher and more frequent doses of the drug to satiate a craving. Users also tend to develop severe depression and personality disorders, along with the loss of brain white matter, which affects decision-making, behavior control, and responses to stressful situations.

Street names: O, Big O, Ope, Aunti, Aunti Emma, Black Pill, Chandu, Chinese Molasses, Chinese Tobacco, Dopium, Dream, Hop/Hops, Midnight Oil, Mira, Zero.

Acute Effects: euphoria, drowsiness, impaired coordination, dizziness, confusion, sedation, inability to feel pain, feeling of heaviness in the body, slowed or arrested breathing.

Health Risks: constipation, heart infection, hepatitis, HIV, addiction, and fatal overdose.

Withdrawal - Opioid withdrawal symptoms are characterized by nausea/vomiting, lacrimation, rhinorrhoea, diarrhea, yawning, sweating, insomnia, dilated pupils, piloerection, chills, dysphoric mood, fever, and life-threatening delirium.

Some opium is heavily contaminated with lead, especially any circulated from 2016 to the present. Lead poisoning can cause learning disabilities, hyperactivity, irritability, headache, memory loss, pain, and fatigue.

Opioid withdrawal delirium is classified in the DSM-5 as a Neurocognitive Disorder (American Psychiatric Association, 2013).

Cocaine

Type: Stimulant
DEA Schedule II Drug
Snorted, Smoked, Absorbed, or Injected

A recreational street drug used in a binge and crash pattern to promote alertness and excitability, artificially speeding up the body and mind. Cocaine is also used to intensify or counteract the effects of sedative drugs. Many individuals use cocaine to help manage symptoms of another mental illness like bipolar disorder, depression, or eating disorders. Cocaine artificially fills empty emotional voids, but long-term cocaine use changes the structure and function of the brain, leading to bizarre, violent, or erratic behavior, and loss of contact with reality.

Street names: Coke, Blow, Bump, C, Candy, Charlie, Crack, Flake, Rock, Snow, Powder, Toot.

Acute Effects: increased heart rate, blood pressure, body temperature, and metabolism; irritability, feelings of exhilaration, increased energy, mental alertness, tremors, reduced appetite, anxiety, panic, paranoia, violent behavior, psychosis.

Health Risks: weight loss, insomnia, headaches, stroke, heart attack, seizures, addiction, nasal damage from snorting, and infection or death of bowel tissue from decreased blood flow. Additionally, a risk of HIV, hepatitis, and infectious disease from shared needles or straws.

Withdrawal - Very unpleasant, but rarely serious unless complicated by suicidal ideation.

Symptoms tend to last only one or two weeks and include depression, anxiety, inability to feel pleasure, exhaustion, challenges in concentration, intense cravings, body aches, pain, tremors, shakiness, chills, vertigo, and muscle twitches.

Methamphetamine

Type: Stimulant
DEA Schedule II Drug
Smoked, Snorted, Ingested, Absorbed, or Injected

An extremely addictive stimulant that disrupts dopamine levels in the brain. It generally resembles glass fragments, dissolves in water or alcohol, and is illegally manufactured from medications intended to treat ADHD, obesity, and congestion. There is a great risk of severe, sometimes permanent, changes in the body and brain with heavy use or high doses of this drug. Many people use meth to feel more confident or to feel energized, but the drug often induces nervousness, agitation, and anxiety attacks. Crystal meth induces a fight-or-flight response, accelerating brain and body functions, and muting signals such as hunger, thirst, or the need for sleep. The powerful dopamine flood, or rush, people experience from using the drug causes addiction right from the start.

Street names: Crystal, Meth, Ice, Tina, Glass, Shards, Blue, Crank, Chalk, Go Fast, Whizz, Speed, Biker's Coffee.

Acute Effects: Increased heart rate, blood pressure, body temperature, metabolism, irritability, feelings of exhilaration, increased energy, mental alertness, tremors, reduced appetite, anxiety, panic, paranoia, violent behavior, psychosis.

Health Risks: severe weight loss, severe dental problems, skin sores, insomnia, stroke, cardiac or cardiovascular complications, seizures, addiction, and severe psychological problems. Methamphetamine has an infamous association with impulsive and aggressive sex, leading to HIV, STIs, and internal injuries.

Withdrawal - As Meth wears off people feel anxious, tired, or depressed. Withdrawal from meth is difficult because extreme cravings, increased appetite, hallucinations, and delusions are common.

MDMA

(Methylenedioxymethamphetamine)
Type: Hallucinogen (Stimulant)
DEA Schedule I Drug
Ingested, Snorted, or Injected

Ecstasy is the common name for this illegal synthetic drug, which speeds up the workings of the central nervous system and alters the perception of reality. MDMA is a psychoactive drug primarily used as a recreational, or club drug. People use this drug to feel euphoric, energized, open, accepting, unafraid, and more connected to the people around them. By releasing large amounts of serotonin, MDMA causes the brain to become significantly depleted of this important neurotransmitter, contributing to the negative psychological aftereffects that people may experience for several days after taking MDMA (NIDA, 2017). Serotonin plays a vital role in regulating mood, sleep, pain, appetite, and behavior.

Street names: Ecstasy, E, Molly (molecular), XTC, Adam, Stacy, Clarity, Eve, Lover's Speed, Essence, and more.

Acute Effects: mild hallucinogenic effects, increased tactile sensitivity, empathic feelings, lowered inhibitions, anxiety, chills, sweating, teeth clenching, muscle cramping.

Health Risks: sleep disturbances, depression, impaired memory, hyperthermia (over-heating), hyponatremia (over-hydrating), and addiction. Mixing this drug with alcohol and/or other drugs can be fatal. MDMA is often adulterated with bath salts, meth, amphetamine, ketamine, or cough medicine.

Withdrawal – As levels of dopamine, serotonin, and norepinephrine drop, users often feel fatigued, depressed, anxious, impulsive, and irritable. In some cases, they become aggressive, have difficulty sleeping, depressed appetite, and trouble concentrating and remembering things.

Mescaline

(Synthetic phenethylamine)
Type: Hallucinogen (Stimulant)
DEA Schedule I Drug
Ingested or Smoked

A naturally occurring psychedelic known for its hallucinogenic effects, which are comparable to those of LSD, DMT, and psilocybin. Mescaline occurs naturally in the peyote cactus, the San Pedro cactus, the Peruvian torch, and other members of the cactus plant family. It is also largely produced in a synthetic phenethylamine form. Synthetic versions of this drug have a molecular similarity to adrenaline, and are structurally related to amphetamine.

Mescaline binds to virtually all serotonin receptors in the brain, producing psychedelic effects, and tends to bind with dopamine receptors, either as a selective reuptake inhibitor or as a dopamine receptor agonist.

Street names: Peyote, Buttons, Cactus, Mesc, Peyoto.

Acute Effects: heatstroke, racing heart, high blood pressure, loss of appetite, sweating, insomnia, numbness, dizziness, tremors, impulsive behavior, shifts in emotion, and acute psychosis.

Health Risks: anxiety, memory loss, tremors, flashbacks, seizures, traumatizing hallucinations, and psychosis.

Withdrawal - Mescaline is psychologically addictive, can induce hallucinogen persisting perception disorder, and may cause stimulant-like withdrawal symptoms.

WARNING: 25I-NBOMe is an especially risky substance to watch out for with mescaline.

2C-B is another psychedelic drug derivative that is structurally similar to mescaline, which is widely available on the Internet.

25I-NBOMe

(Synthetic phenethylamine)
Type: Hallucinogen (Stimulant)
DEA Schedule I Drug
Absorbed, Injected, Smoked, Vaporized, or Snorted

N-BOMe, commonly referred to as "N-bomb" or "Smiles," is a powerful synthetic hallucinogen sold as an alternative to LSD or mescaline. 25I-NBOMe is used in biochemistry research for mapping the brain's usage of the type 2A serotonin receptor, and it has made its way into the recreational drug using community. It creates an hallucinogenic effect similar to LSD, but at extremely small dosages. A dose of 750 micrograms, which is considered an average to high dose, is about the size of six small grains of regular table salt. It only takes a few grains to produce an effect, and it is extremely easy to overdose when taking this drug, with sometimes-fatal consequences.

Street names: 25I, 25C, 25B, BOM-CI or Cimbi-5, Dime, GNOME, Legal Acid, N-bomb, New Nexus, Smiles, Solaris.

Acute Effects: confusion, paranoia, insomnia, chaotic excitement, uncontrollable laughing, flushing, extreme panic, racing heart, fever, nausea, agitation, numbness, loss of fine motor skills, severe disorientation, violent outbursts, and frightening hallucinations.

Health Risks: psychosis, violent aggression, suicidal thoughts, brain damage, organ damage, seizures, and possible death.

Withdrawal - Users report the negative effects and after-effects of the drug are worse than that of LSD. This drug also mimics the withdrawal symptoms of methamphetamine.

WARNING: Dealers sell it as other less potent hallucinogens, and users take a known normal dose, resulting in a fatal overdose. N-bomb is extremely toxic, and requires protective gear while handling it.

Spice (K2)

(Synthetic cannabinoids)
Type: Hallucinogen (Stimulant)
DEA Schedule I Drug
Smoked or Vaporized

Synthetic cannabinoids are misleadingly marketed as safe and legal alternatives. They are not safe, and affect the brain much more powerfully than marijuana. A 2019 study of the behavioral, physiological, cognitive, and subjective experiences caused by synthetic cannabis products in humans showed that (Spice) is in fact (five times) more potent than THC. Teens and adolescents often experiment with this drug, to get high, because it is easier to obtain than marijuana. Spice products are labeled **not for human consumption**. Some of these synthesized compounds bind much more strongly to THC receptors than regular marijuana, which leads to more powerful, unpredictable, and dangerous effects.

Labels: Clone, K2, Spice, Joker, Black Mamba, Kush, Kronic, and hundreds of other brand names marketed as *incense*.

Acute Effects: altered perception, anxiety, excessive sweating, confusion, extreme anxiety, extreme paranoia, hallucinations, extreme aggression, seizures, and heart attacks.

Health Risks: bruising, excessive bleeding, back or stomach pain, loss of consciousness, flash backs, and memory loss.

Withdrawal – emotional distress, anxiety, depression, irritability, headaches, concentration issues, restlessness, sweating, nausea, excessive vomiting, tremors, insomnia, nightmares, severe cravings, suicidal thoughts, and self-harm.

WARNING: Manufacturers contaminate Spice products with blood thinners and rat poison, which causes severe bleeding, coma or death.

LSD

(Lysergic acid diethylamide)
Type: Hallucinogen
DEA Schedule I Drug
Ingested or Absorbed

LSD is an extremely potent and mood-altering psychedelic. It is manufactured from the ergot fungus that grows on rye and other grains. It is odorless, colorless, and has a slightly bitter taste. People use LSD as a recreational drug, for spiritual reasons, or for a complete disconnection from reality. Professor Jack Cohen, a mathematical biologist, theorized that the kaleidoscope visual hallucinations that users experience while on the drug derive from the innate tendency of the brain to make patterns when it becomes unstable. LSD is lethal in high doses, and causes devastating effects when people dose unknowingly, or if they already struggle with a mental disorder.

Street names: Acid, Blotter, Doses, Microdot, Tab, Yellow Sunshine, California Sunshine, Heavenly Blue, Looney Tunes, and more.

Acute Effects: altered thoughts, feelings, and awareness of one's surrounding, see or hear things that do not exist, dilated pupils, increased blood pressure, and increased body temperature, impulsive behavior, shifts in emotion.

Effects typically begin within 30 minutes and can last for up to 12 hours, depending on purity and dosage.

Health Risks: anxiety, memory loss, tremors, flashbacks, and Hallucinogen Persisting Perception Disorder (HPPD). At least five percent of users experience flashbacks, a brief, spontaneous return of an hallucinogenic effect that can occur weeks, or even months later.

Withdrawal - Physical withdrawal symptoms are uncomfortable, and continued LSD use can develop into a psychological dependency.

DMT

(N-dimethyltryptamine)
Type: Hallucinogen
DEA Schedule I Drug
Smoked, Snorted, or Brewed

DMT is a powerful psychoactive substance that can cause a number of mental and physical **side effects**. People are drawn to it because they believe it may give them a mystical near-death or out-of-body experience. Dr. Rick Strassman explains, "There are data suggesting urinary DMT rises in psychotic patients when their psychosis is worse." DMT has negative interactions with a range of prescription and over-the-counter medications, as well as most other drugs.

Street names: Ayahuasca, Dimitri, Fantasia, Businessman's Trip, Spiritual Molecule, 45-minute Psychosis.

Acute Effects: racing heart, increased blood pressure, visual disturbances, dizziness, dilated pupils, agitation, confusion, paranoia, rapid rhythmic eye movements, chest pain or tightness, diarrhea, nausea or vomiting.

Health Risks: anxiety, tremors, numbness, memory loss, flashbacks, loss of coordination, seizures, respiratory arrest, and possible coma. Like other hallucinogenic drugs, DMT may cause persistent psychosis and hallucinogen persisting perception disorder (HPPD).

Withdrawal - Uncomfortable, psychological symptoms, HPPD.

WARNING: DMT can result in high levels of the neurotransmitter serotonin. This can lead to a potentially life threatening condition called Serotonin Syndrome Disorder. People who use DMT while taking antidepressants, especially monoamine oxidase inhibitors (MAOIs), have a higher risk for developing this condition. Seek immediate medical attention for Serotonin Syndrome.

Magic Mushrooms

(Psilocybin)
Type: Hallucinogen
DEA Schedule I Drug
Ingested or Smoked

Mushrooms contain a compound called psilocybin, a chemical that activates serotonin receptors in the brain, triggering vivid hallucinations, a sense of euphoria, and changes in perception of space and time. Since they are found growing in the wild, many people mistake this drug as a safe alternative to harder drugs. It is important to understand that studies done on psilocybin are done in controlled environments with a controlled dosage. Self-medicating with this drug, or using it recreationally with other drugs can and does produce wildly different outcomes.

As with any powerful hallucinogen, there is a great risk that the drug will bring to light, or worsen, any underlying mental health problems and disorders. Many users experience enjoyable sensations, while others experience terrifying thoughts, anxiety, and fears of insanity, death, or losing control. A person using magic mushrooms is often unable to discern what is fantasy and what is reality.

Street names: Caps, Magic Mushrooms, Shrooms. Many slang terms derive from the different drugs mixed with the mushrooms.

Acute Effects: nausea, euphoria, waves of intoxication, sensory distortion, altered perception, nervousness, and paranoia.

Health Risks: disturbing hallucinations, anxiety, panic, flashbacks, and hallucinogen persisting perception disorder.

Withdrawal – Psilocybin is psychologically addictive, causing lasting changes to the brain and mental health issues.

Salvia Divinorium

(Salvinorin A)
Type: Hallucinogen (Opioid)
DEA Unscheduled - Drug of Concern - FDA Warning
Smoked, Vaporized, or Chewed

Salvia is an herbal mint plant and a natural occurring hallucinogen that is native to Mexico. It is a member of the sage family. People use it as a recreational drug. There are concerns that salvia may affect a person's thinking, choices, and mental health. Classified as a dissociative drug, salvia divinorum affects the brain differently. Salvinorin-A changes the signaling process of nerve cells in the brain by attaching to kappa opioid receptors. These receptors are different from those that are activated by opiates, such as morphine and heroin. The KOR seems to play a key role in regulating human perception. Salvia may also influence dopamine receptors in the brain.

Street names: Magic Mint, Sally-D, Diviner's Sage, Seer's Sage, Ska Maria Pastora, Shepherdess's Herb, Lady Sally, Purple Sticky, and Incense Special.

Acute Effects: nausea, tiredness, dizziness, lack of coordination, difficulty concentrating, confusion, slurred speech, flushing, memory loss, hallucinations, spatio-temporal dislocation, and uncontrollable laughter, fear, or panic.

*Spatio-temporal dislocation is where the user feels transported to an alternative time and place, or has a feeling of being in several locations at once. Disruption of space and time can be a frightening experience and can lead to serious psychotic disturbances in vulnerable people.

Withdrawal - The long-term effects are not known. However, studies with animals showed that salvia harms learning and memory.

PCP & Analogs

(Phencyclidine)
Type: Dissociative (Anesthetic)
DEA Schedule II Drug
Injected, Snorted, Smoked, or Ingested

PCP was developed in the 1950s as a surgical anesthetic, but the drug was soon discontinued after it was found to cause agitation, mania, distorted reality, and irrational thinking. This type of drug affects multiple neurotransmitter systems in the brain. It inhibits the reuptake of dopamine, norepinephrine, and serotonin. PCP also inhibits the action of glutamate by blocking receptors that are responsible for pain sensation, emotions, learning, and memory functions. Interrupting these receptors allows the brain to disconnect from reality. In higher doses, however, it may also excite these receptors. The induced sense of super strength, invulnerability, and inability to feel pain leads to serious injury. Vulnerable users may develop a type of psychosis similar to schizophrenia. Users are often brought to emergency rooms because of the drug's severe psychological effects and violent or suicidal behaviors.

Street names: Angel Dust, Wack, Embalming Fluid, Killer Weed, Elephant Tranquilizer, Hog, Ozone, Peace Pill, Super Grass, Rocket Fuel, and more.

Acute Effects: euphoria, dissociation from reality, numbness, loss of coordination, anxiety, agitation, mood swings, confusion, slurred speech, blank stare, stupor, combativeness, aggression, bizarre behavior, and schizophrenia-like delusions.

Health Risks: suicidal thoughts, combative or violent behavior, increased heart rate, visual distortions, psychosis, seizures, muscle damage, chest pain, hypertension, serious injury or death.

Withdrawal – Sudden detox from PCP results in severe cravings and depression. Hospitalization is often necessary.

Ketamine

Type: Dissociative (Anesthetic)
DEA Schedule III Drug
Injected, Snorted, Ingested, or Smoked

Ketamine is a medication mainly used for starting and maintaining anesthesia, and it is illegal to use it recreationally. It induces a trance-like state while providing pain relief, sedation, and memory loss. As a medication, it is sometimes prescribed for chronic pain, depression, and intensive care sedation.

Ketamine and PCP are both dissociative anesthetic drugs, which distort perception of sight and sound, and produce feelings of detachment from the environment and self. The liquid form of ketamine is often stolen from veterinary offices and then sold as a recreational drug. Ketamine users develop deep cravings, and at high doses, users experience an out of body effect or near-death experience.

Street names: Ketalar SV, Cat Valium, K, Special K, Vitamin K.

Acute Effects: numbness, dream-like feeling, blurred/double vision, jerky movements, dizziness, drowsiness, nausea, vomiting, loss of appetite, depression, severe confusion, delusions, and hallucinations.

Health Risks: loss of consciousness, insomnia, extreme fear, increased heart rate and blood pressure, serious bladder problems, anorexia, seizures, potentially fatal respiratory problems, coma, possible death.

Withdrawal - Frequent or chronic Ketamine users develop a tolerance to the drug, along with a psychological dependence, and very strong cravings when not taking the drug.

WARNING: Ketamine induces a detached and dreamlike state, making it difficult to move and vulnerable to victimization, such as date rape.

Rohypnol

(Flunitrazepam)
Type: Benzodiazepine (Sedative-Hypnotic)
DEA Schedule IV Drug
Ingested, Injected, Snorted, or Smoked

Rohypnol is still legal in many countries as a medication to treat severe insomnia and to assist with anesthesia in surgery. It became synonymous with sexual assault, but many people today abuse it simply for recreation. Rohypnol is a tranquilizer that is ten times more potent than Valium, and affects the brain immediately once it enters the body. It diminishes the ability to make logical decisions, which leads to risky behavior. Users often describe the effects as *paralyzing*, and can last for 8 to 12 hours. Afterwards, memory is impaired and they cannot recall anything from the experience.

Street names: Roofies, Forget-me Pill, Mexican Valium, R2, Roche, La Rocha, Roofinol, Rope, Rophies, and more.

Acute Effects: sedation, muscle relaxation, confusion, memory loss, dizziness, emphatic feelings, and lowered inhibitions.

Health Risks: Rohypnol can cause physical and psychological addiction, loss of muscle control, and blackouts.
Commonly used in sexual assaults.

Withdrawal - Intense withdrawal symptoms such as seizures and psychosis can result when stopping regular use of this drug because the physical dependence is severe. Withdrawal effects are very similar to alcohol withdrawal, such as muscle pain, numbness, tremors, delirium, shock, convulsions, and hallucinations.

WARNING: Rohypnol may be lethal when mixed with alcohol and/or other depressants. Clonazepam is a very similar drug, and is being sold as "roofies" on the streets.

GHB

(Gamma-hydroxybutyrate)
Type: CNS Depressant (Sedative)
DEA Schedule I Drug
Injected, Snorted, or Smoked

GHB is a colorless and tasteless drug that is used illicitly for recreational purposes and infamously for date rape. Manufacturers market it as a growth hormone, a sexual performance enhancer, or a workout enhancement. There seems to be low-dose experimental trials with this drug to treat narcolepsy, alcoholism, and heroin addiction. There are more than 350 known deaths related to GHB intoxication.

GHB is a central nervous system depressant, and users believe that it gives them the relaxing effects of alcohol without the loss of coordination, slurred speech, or a hangover. In higher doses, it can cause someone to fall unconscious, and the effects are amplified when mixed with alcohol, possibly causing unconsciousness within minutes.

Street names: G, Liquid Ecstasy, Georgia Home Boy, Grievous Bodily Harm, Easy Lay, Soap, Scoop, Goop, Liquid X.

Acute Effects: drowsiness, dizziness, nausea, headache, loss of coordination, disorientation, memory lapses, and hallucinations.

Health Risks: lowered temperature, clumsiness, shallow breathing, vomiting, blackouts, unconsciousness, seizures, coma.

Withdrawal – Founder of Project GHB and former LAPD Detective, Trinka Porrata claim, "GHB is harder to quit than Heroin." Symptoms include insomnia, anxiety, tremors, increased heart rate and blood pressure, and psychotic thoughts.

WARNING: Very serious interactions occur when taken with alcohol and/or other depressants.

DXM & Codeine-Based Cough Syrup

(Dextromethorphan)
Type: Dissociative (Anesthetic, Hallucinogen, Opiate/Sedative)
DEA Not Scheduled (DXM)
DEA Sechedule I/II Drug by potency (Codeine)
Ingested: Mixed with Sugar Drinks, Candy, and/or Alcohol

DXM is a cough suppressant, generally sold over-the-counter in syrup, tablet, spray, and lozenge forms are easy to obtain and hide. It is in the morphinan class of medications with sedative, dissociative, and stimulant properties (at lower doses). Taken in high doses, it can produce mind-altering effects similar to PCP and Ketamine. Many cough syrup formulas also contain decongestants, pain relievers, and antihistamines, so the effects of DXM abuse can also include risks of addiction, respiratory distress, seizures, and increased heart rate. Mixing DXM with alcohol carries a high likelihood of addiction and life-threatening symptoms.

Street names: Purple Drank, Sizzurp, Lean, Robotripping, Triple C, Poor Man's PCP, Velvet, Skittles, Rojo, Dex, Orange Crush, Red Devils.

Acute Effects: mild euphoria, agitation, dissociation and confusion, slurred speech, muscle twitch, dizziness, distorted visual perceptions.

Health Risks: panic, mania, tremors, memory loss, vivid nightmares, delusions, hallucinations, paranoia, disorientation, irrational sense of flying, liver damage, violent behaviors, suicide.

Withdrawal - Extremely uncomfortable with restlessness, insomnia, bone or muscle aches, cold flashes, diarrhea, vomiting, cravings, and significant weight loss.

DXM abuse can result in toxic psychosis, which is characterized by confusion and losing contact with reality. Individuals experiencing substance-induced psychosis have trouble recognizing their environment and communicating with others.

Cathinones (Bath Salts)

Type: Synthetic Stimulants
DEA Temporarily Banned Ingredients
Injected, Snorted, Ingested, or Smoked

Synthetic cathinone products marketed as "bath salts" should not be confused with products such as Epsom salts that people use during bathing. These bathing products have no mind-altering ingredients.

The street drugs are cheap substitutes for other stimulants such as methamphetamine and cocaine. Drugs such as MDMA (Molly) often contain these synthetic cathinones. For example, hundreds of MDMA (Ecstasy) capsules tested in two South Florida crime labs in 2012 contained methylone, a dangerous synthetic cathinone. Synthetic cathinones are unregulated psychoactive mind-altering substances with no legitimate medical use. They are introduced and reintroduced into the market in quick succession to dodge or hinder law enforcement efforts to address their manufacture and sale.

Labels: Bliss, Cloud Nine, Ivory, Wave, Vanilla Sky, White Lightning.

Acute Effects: agitation, increased friendliness, increased sex drive.

Health Risks: dehydration, breakdown of skeletal muscle tissue, suicidal thoughts, confusion, panic attacks, combative or violent behavior, increased heart rate, excited delirium, hallucinations, psychosis, chest pain, kidney failure, serious injury or death.

Withdrawal - Taking synthetic cathinones can cause strong withdrawal symptoms that include depression, anxiety, tremors, problems sleeping, and paranoia. Users also report an intense and uncontrollable urge to take the drug again.

Inhalants

Type: Other Compound
DEA Not Scheduled
Inhaled

Of the more than 1,000 household products that could be abused as inhalants, most often they are shoe polish, glue, toluene, gasoline, lighter fluid, nitrous oxide (whippets), spray paint, correction fluid, cleaning fluid, amyl nitrite (poppers), locker room deodorizers (rush), and lacquer thinner, spray paint, and paint solvents.

The effects are similar to anesthetics, which slow down the body's functions. After an initial high and loss of inhibition comes drowsiness, light-headedness, and agitation. Chemicals are rapidly absorbed through the lungs into the bloodstream and quickly reach the brain and other organs, sometimes causing irreversible physical and mental damage.

Users inhale the chemical vapors directly from open containers (sniffing) or breathe the fumes from rags soaked in chemicals (huffing). Some people spray the substance directly into their nose or mouth, or pour it onto their collar, sleeves, or cuffs so they can sniff them periodically. The user also may inhale fumes from substances inside a paper or plastic bag. "Bagging" in a closed area greatly increases the chances of suffocation.

Poppers and *whippets* sold at concerts and dance clubs, are composed of poisonous chemicals that can permanently damage the body and brain.

Street names: laughing gas, poppers, snappers, whippets, rush.

Acute Effects: stimulation, loss of inhibition, headache, nausea, vomiting, slurred speech, loss of motor coordination, wheezing.

Health Risks: cramps, muscle weakness, depression, memory impairment, damage to cardiovascular and nervous systems, unconsciousness, and sudden death.

Anabolic Steroids

Type: Synthetic Hormones
DEA Schedule III Drug (some exempt)
Injected, Absorbed, Ingested, Implanted

Anabolic steroids are used illegally to increase muscle, decrease fat, and enhance athletic performance and body appearance. People who use steroids to enhance their appearance may suffer from muscle dysmorphia or an abnormal perception of their own body. Males may think that they are perpetually too small and weak, and females may think of themselves as fat, even though those perceptions might not actually be true.

Some physicians believe that the decreased testosterone levels that occurs normally with aging is an indication for replacement therapy with anabolic steroids, but their use in otherwise healthy older patients is still controversial because of the potential **serious side effects**.

Examples of anabolic steroids:

- Testosterone (Axiron, Androgel, Fortesta, Testopel, Striant, Delatestryl, Testim, Androderm)
- Androstenedione
- Stanozolol (Winstrol)
- Nandrolone (Deca-Durabolin)
- Methandrosteolone (Dianabol)
- Depo-Provera

Anabolic steroids used as performance-enhancing drugs increase the ability to do work and exercise by abnormally stimulating muscle growth, power, and aerobic capacity. This increased function comes with a cost of potentially life-threatening **side effects**. The complications of steroid abuse are a result of excess testosterone affecting almost all the organ systems in the body. Some of effects are reversible and decrease when the drug abuse stops, while others are permanent and irreversible.

In males, the excess steroid suppresses the normal testosterone production in the body. This can lead to shrunken testicles and decreased sperm count, baldness, and breast development (gynecomastia).

In females, anabolic steroid abuse can lead to masculinization with loss of body fat and breast size, swelling of the clitoris (which may be permanent and not resolve, even if a woman stops using steroids), deepening of the voice, and the development of facial and body hair.

Life-threatening Side Effects include: heart attack and stroke, the risk of forming blood clots, liver cancer, and liver failure.

Acute Effects: acne, fluid retention, rapid weight gain, increased blood pressure and cholesterol levels, insomnia, headaches, reduced sexual functioning, increase in muscle size, swelling of feet and ankles.

Psychiatric and psychological complications include manic behavior and psychosis, including hallucinations and delusions. Aggressive behavior is very common and known as '**roid rage**'.

Muscle growth can occur quickly causing stress on the tendons that attach the muscle to bone, so there is a risk for tendon rupture. Anabolic steroids can also increase bone production, especially in the skull and face. Teeth can splay apart as the maxilla and mandible grow, along with an overgrowth of the forehead, giving an "Incredible Hulk" appearance.

Withdrawal - mood swings, fatigue, restlessness, loss of appetite, insomnia, reduced sex drive, and steroid cravings.

The most dangerous of the withdrawal symptoms is depression, because it sometimes leads to suicide attempts. If left untreated, some depressive symptoms associated with anabolic steroid withdrawal have been known to persist for a year or more after the abuser stops taking the drugs.

Street names: roids, juice, gym, candy, pumpers.

Part Two: Prescription Drugs

A drug-free society or freedom from **ALL** drugs?

Polypharmacy: the simultaneous use of 5 or more drugs to treat a single ailment or condition.

Hyperpolypharmacy: the simultaneous use of 10 or more drugs to treat a single ailment or condition.

In our 'take a pill' over-medicating culture, we've gotten to the point where doctors have to prescribe more drugs just to treat the **side-effects** of other prescriptions.

The Opiate receptor for Trauma Pain Management

Opiates such as morphine have long been known to effectively reduce pain. In 1974, Candace Pert discovered that the brain has its own opiate receptor, the cellular binding site for endorphins. This provides evidence that the brain must produce something on its own that is akin to drugs like morphine.

Dr. Pert's discovery of opiate-like chemicals produced in the body that control pain, immune responses, and other bodily functions was an invaluable milestone. Prior to the opiate receptor discovery, scientists knew little about opiate drugs and how they affected the brain. It was merely known that opiates acted on specific neurons, and opiate drugs that blocked their action shared a similar molecular structure. This new knowledge led to the identification of **endorphins** which have the same actions as pain management drugs.

In her book, *Molecules of Emotion - The SSRI Saga* (1997), Dr. Pert stated:

> "I am alarmed at the monster that Johns Hopkins neuroscientist Solomon Snyder and I created when we discovered the simple binding assay for drug receptors 25 years ago. The public is being misinformed about the precision of these selective serotonin-up-take inhibitors when the medical profession oversimplifies their action in the brain and ignores the body as if it exists merely to carry the head around! These molecules of emotion regulate every aspect of our physiology. A new paradigm has evolved, with implications that life-style changes such as diet and exercise offer profound, safe, and natural mood elevation."

Stop the Shootings – In 1998, Dr. Pert pointed out that in all of the school shootings, the shooter had been on psychotropic medications. Single and mass shootings continue today with adults, teens, and children on a daily basis. Has no one paid attention to her warning?

Opioids (Narcotics)

Type: Highly Addictive
DEA Schedule II Drugs
Pills, Lozenges, Lollipops, Patches, Sprays, or Injected

Opioids bind to and activate opiate receptors in many areas of the brain, spinal cord, and other organs in the body, especially those involved in feelings of pain and pleasure. Once activated, receptors block pain signals sent from the brain to the body, which releases large amounts of dopamine throughout the body. This unnatural and immediate dopamine release intensely reinforces the act of taking the drug, making the user want to repeat the experience. Prolonged use of opioid medication causes the body to become desensitized to the effects. Over time, the brain becomes dependant on the drug and thinks it needs more and more of the drug to achieve the same effect. This can be very dangerous and increases the risk of accidental overdose. Many people become dependent on these drugs in order to avoid pain or withdrawal symptoms. In some cases, people don't even realize that they've become dependent. They may mistake withdrawal for symptoms of the flu or another condition. Opioids are highly addictive and easily misused and abused, making overdose and death very common.

Prescribed For: chronic, persistent or severe pain.

Acute Effects: sleepiness, constipation, nausea, pain relief.

Side Effects: physical dependency & addiction, sudden mental or mood changes, anxiety, depression, severe drowsiness, dizziness, loss of appetite, confusion, weight loss, shallow breathing, slowed heart rate, hallucinations, loss of consciousness.

Withdrawal (Severe) - intense drug cravings, flu-like symptoms, agitation, anxiety, insomnia, goose bumps, vision problems, abdominal pain, vomiting, diarrhea, excessive sweating, thoughts of suicide, tremors (shaking), rapid heartbeat, high blood pressure, seizures.

WARNING: **Very serious interactions** occur when taken with alcohol and/or other depressants.

*Opioid medications combined with Acetaminophen may cause circulatory failure, and rapid, shallow breathing—often causing death.

**Patients taking Medication Assisted Therapy drugs should continue to take these medicines as prescribed. Do not stop taking prescribed medicines without first talking to a health care professional. Do not take non-prescribed benzodiazcpines or other sedatives or use alcohol when taking MAT drugs because the combined use increases the possibility of harm, including overdose and death.

COMMON OPIOID MEDICATIONS

Darvocet® (dextropropoxyphene)
Banned in 2010 as a dangerous combined opiate analgesic due to adverse cardiotoxicity and other common fatal effects.

Fentanyl (Duragesic®, Abstral®, Ionsys®)
50–100 times more potent than morphine; death is likely, and it is known to be combined with Heroin.

**Carfentanyl is 10,000 times more potent than morphine, and 100 times stronger than fentanyl.

Lorcet® (hydrocodone/acetaminophen)
An immediate-release pain reliever combining a synthetic opiate with Acetaminophen. High doses can be toxic to the liver when used over a length of time.

Lortab® (hydrocodone/acetaminophen)
Another brand name for Vicodin.

Lucemyra® (lofexidine)

Lucemyra is used to reduce opioid withdrawal symptoms. It blocks the release of norepinephrine, a hormone similar to adrenaline, which contributes to opioid withdrawal symptoms. **Warning:** this drug can cause serious damage in the heart and blood vessels.

Methadone (Diskets®, Methadone Intensol, Methadose®)

A long-acting synthetic opioid, commonly referred to as an opioid replacement therapy for addiction to heroin and other opiates. It is actually a replacement addiction.

Methadone Raises Risk of Respiratory Depression and QT Interval Prolongation

Methadone has a **black box warning** for increasing the risk of respiratory depression and QT interval prolongation. The package labeling states that cardiac and respiratory death has been reported during methadone initiation and conversion from other opioid agonists. Respiratory depression is the chief hazard associated with methadone administration.

The drug's peak respiratory depressant effects typically occur after administration and persist longer than its peak analgesic effects, particularly in the early dosing period. These characteristics can contribute to cases of drug overdose, particularly during treatment initiation and dose titration.

In addition, cases of QT interval prolongation and serious arrhythmia have been observed during methadone treatment. Most cases involve patients who were treated for pain with large, multiple daily doses of methadone, although cases have also been reported in patients receiving doses commonly used for maintenance treatment of opioid addiction. "Methadone should only be initiated if the drug's potential analgesic or palliative care benefit outweighs the risks." -- The FDA.

Morphine (MorphaBond ER®, Arymo ER®, Infumorph P/F®)
An opiate sourced from the straw of opium poppy plants and has been used for pain relief since the 1900s. 70% of the morphine produced today is used to make synthetic opiates such as Oxycodone.

Norco® (hydrocodone/acetaminophen)
Another brand name for Vicodin.

Oxycontin® (oxycodone)
An opioid analgesic narcotic that can cause respiratory distress and death when taken in high doses or when combined with other substances, especially alcohol.

Percocet® (oxycodone/acetaminophen)
A habit-forming synthetic opioid approved by FDA in 1999 and since has been the focus by DEA to reduce the soaring number of overdose deaths and emergency room visits.

Suboxone® (buprenorphine)
Buprenorphine is a partial opioid agonist. It is also a Controlled substance with a High risk for addiction and dependence. **Suboxone can cause respiratory distress and death when taken in high doses or when combined with other substances, especially alcohol.** As with all interventions in medicine, buprenorphine treatment for narcotic addiction has a clinically fluctuating risk/benefit equation that must be continually monitored.

Ultram® (tramadol)
The extended-release form is for around-the-clock treatment of pain, and is **not** for use on an as-needed basis for pain.

Vicodin® (hydrocodone)
A commly abused opioid analgesic narcotic.

Antidepressants (SSRI, SNRI, SARI, NDRI, Tetracyclic, TCA, MAOI)

Primarily prescribed to manage depression, but they are often used to treat a wide range of mental disorders. There is no scientific evidence that a person suffering anxiety or depression has a chemical imbalance. The imbalance occurs when they take psychiatric drugs. Antidepressants can cause mania and aggression, possibly leading to criminal acts of violence. The sheer number of murders (and homicidal thoughts) now linked to antidepressant medications is truly overwhelming.

Antidepressant chemicals create dramatic changes in the brain. Changes in the functional structure of the brain have been observed after a single dose, and it is noted that even an unadulterated human brain is not fully developed until a person reaches at least age 25.

> ## FDA Black Box Warning:
> Use may increase suicidal thoughts or actions in some children, teenagers, or young adults within the first few months of treatment, when a dose is changed, or if discontinued.

- Amitriptyline
- Celexa® (citalopram)
- Cymbalta® (duloxetine)
- Desyrel® (trazodone)
- Effexor® (venlafaxine)
- Lexapro® (escitalopram)
- Paxil® (paroxetine)
- Prozac® (fluoxetine)
- Remeron® (mirtazapine)
- Wellbutrin® (bupropion)
- Zoloft® (sertraline)
- Viibryd® (vilazodone)

Professional Titration Required - Stopping these meds abruptly can cause serious symptoms such as anxiety, irritability, high or low mood, feeling restless, changes in sleep habits, headache, sweating, nausea, dizziness, electric shock-like sensations, shaking, or confusion.

Each type of antidepressant will have its own unique properties, and there are seven 'subclasses' of antidepressants that have different 'mechanisms of action' of how they work. SSRI medications interrupt and block the normal transmission of serotonin along the nerve channels. This interruption can often result in a build-up in the nerve synapses. Eventually, the blocked neurotransmitters degrade, which may lead to a serotonin deficit and worsened symptoms.

Neurotransmitters are designed to work together, not independently of each other. When one neurotransmitter is artificially changed, others try to compensate or regain a semblance of balance. Science has found that over stimulating receptor sites with SSRIs will cause the receptors to become desensitized, leaving the brain dependent on the drug, and cannot function without the higher levels of stimulating serotonin.

Side Effects & **Withdrawal Symptoms** are common: nausea, vomiting, cramps, diarrhea, appetite loss, vertigo, insomnia, nightmares, flu-like symptoms, extreme anxiety, agitation, panic, suicidal ideation, depression, irritability, anger, mania, mood swings, excessive sweating, flushing, tremors, muscle tension, restless legs, unsteady gait, difficulty controlling speech, and chewing movements.

Sexual Side Effects such as numbness, problems with orgasm, or ejaculatory delay often **do not diminish** over time.

Serotonin Syndrome (SS) otherwise known as Serotonin toxicity, is a life threatening drug-induced condition caused by too much serotonin in the brain. Drug interactions, alcohol use, and medication overdose are the most likely causes of SS. Drugs such as ecstasy, LSD, cocaine, and amphetamines can also cause Serotonin Syndrome.

Toxicity Symptoms include: confusion, delirium, hallucinations, tremors, rapid heart rate, headache, high fever, dilated pupils, dizziness, nausea and vomiting, diarrhea, seizures, heart attack, coma, and death.

Antipsychotics (1st Generation & 2nd Generation)

Also known as neuroleptics or major tranquilizers, these drugs are used in the short-term to manage psychosis and psychotic behaviors (including delusions, hallucinations, paranoia, or disorganized thoughts), primarily observed in schizophrenia and bipolar disorder. People with anxiety and mood disorders are also prescribed antipsychotics in addition to antidepressants or mood stabilizers.

Psychosis is believed to be caused, at least in part, by over-activity of dopamine in the brain, and antipsychotics are thought to work by blocking this dopamine effect. This blocking helps to make the symptoms of psychosis—such as voices and delusions—less commanding and preoccupying, but it does not always make them go away completely. People may still hear voices and have delusions, but they are more able to recognize what isn't real and to focus on other things, such as work, school or family.

Antipsychotic medications can cause unpleasant side-effects, especially when the symptoms are severe and a higher dose of medication is prescribed. Most side-effects dissipate after titrating off the drug, but the risk of **Antipsychotic-Induced Movement Disorders** is real and can be permanent.

Some people accept the **side-effects** as a trade-off for the relief these drugs can bring. Others find the side-effects distressing and may choose not to take the medication. **Never** stop taking these medications abruptly.

> **Movement Effects:** Tremors, muscle stiffness and tics can occur. The higher the dose, the more severe these effects. The risk of these effects may be lower with the second generation medications than with the older drugs.

> **Dizziness:** Feelings of dizziness and fainting may occur, especially when getting up from a sitting or lying position.

Weight Gain: Some of the second generation drugs are thought to affect people's sense of having had enough to eat. They can also be sedating. These two effects can result in weight gain, which can increase a person's risk of diabetes and heart disease.

Diabetes: Schizophrenia is a risk factor for diabetes. Antipsychotic drugs can increase this risk.

Agitation and Sedation: Some people feel "wired" and unable to stop moving when taking antipsychotics. This effect may be mistaken for a worsening of illness rather than a side-effect of the medication. These same drugs can also have the opposite effect, making people feel tired. Some people may feel either wired or tired, and some may feel both at the same time.

Tardive Dyskinesia: Each year that a person takes antipsychotic medication, there is a 5% chance of developing tardive dyskinesia (TD), a condition that causes people to have repetitive involuntary movements. The risk of TD is highest with the first generation antipsychotics, although it can occur with the second generation drugs. TD can worsen when the medication is discontinued and can be permanent.

Neuroleptic Malignant Syndrome: Rare but serious complication usually associated with the use of high doses of typical antipsychotics early in treatment. Signs include fever, muscle stiffness and delirium.

Noted Side Effects: Movements of the jaw, lips, and tongue (TD); Sexual problems (hormonal changes); Sleepiness and slowness; Metabolic changes; Interrupted breathing during sleep; Constipation; Dry mouth; Blurred vision; Drooling; Compulsive behaviors; Delusions; Thoughts of Suicide.

Abilify® (aripiprazole)
A 2nd-generation atypical psychotic medication used in the treatment of adult schizophrenia, bipolar disorder, Tourette syndrome, and in young children (age restrictions) presenting symptoms of autistic spectrum disorder (temper tantrums, mood swings, and aggression).

Clozaril® (clozapine)
Clozaril is often prescribed only after other antipsychotics did not work or caused severe side effects.

Caplyta® (lumateperone)
The FDA recently approved this new brand for adults with schizophrenia.

Depakote® (valproic acid/divalproex sodium)
An anti-seizure drug that can cause paradoxical seizures, which are potentially life-threatening, on abrupt withdrawal from the med. **Serious Side Effects** are dizziness, drowsiness, hair loss, double vision, ringing in the ears, tremor, unsteadiness, depression, and suicidal thoughts.

Fanapt® (iloperidone)
A 2nd generation atypical antipsychotic for schizophrenia in adults. **Serious Side Effects** are dizziness, light-headedness, drooling, trouble swallowing, muscle spasms, interrupted breathing during sleep, fainting, seizures, and trouble breathing.

Geodon® (ziprasidone)
Atypical 2nd-generation antipsychotic available since 2001. Prescribed to treat mood disorders, schizophrenia, and bipolar symptoms. There's a risk of heart damage, along with a rise in blood cholesterol.

Latuda® (lurasidone)
An atypical antipsychotic used to treat schizophrenia and depression associated with bipolar disorder. **Side Effects** include agitation, hostility, confusion, drooling, shaking, weight gain, and thoughts of self-harm.

Lamictal® (lamotrigine)

An anti-convulsive medication used for seizures, and is also prescribed as a maintenance drug to delay reoccurring bipolar episodes of depression, mania, and hypomania. Lamictal has a **black box warning** for causing cases of life-threatening serious rashes, including Stevens-Johnson syndrome, toxic epidermal necrolysis, and/or rash-related death.

Lithium

Lithium salts such as Lithobid® are prescribed for the treatment of mania, bipolar disorders, depression, and PTSD. Natural lithium supplements are available OTC. **Serious Side Effects** are drowsiness, dizziness, lightheadedness, drop in blood pressure, muscle twitching and uncontrollable movements, weight gain, drooling, trouble swallowing, fainting, and interrupted breathing during sleep.

Risperdal® (risperidone)

An antipsychotic used to treat children (5-16yrs old) diagnosed with autism, patients age 13+ for schizophrenia, and adults and children age 10+ who suffer acute manic mixed episodes of bipolar disorder.

Saphris® (asenapine)

Atypical antipsychotic prescribed to treat the symptoms of schizophrenia and bipolar episodic mania. **Serious Side Effects** are light headedness, drowsiness, dizziness, anxiety, agitation, jitteriness, drooling, trouble swallowing, restlessness, constant need to move, tremor, shuffling walk, stiff muscles, cramping, weight gain, and blood sugar elevation.

Seroquel® (quetiapine)

Atypical antipsychotic for schizophrenia symptoms and mixed bipolar episodes (acute manic and major depressive episodes). **Serious Side Effects** are restlessness/constant need to move, shakiness, mental/mood changes such as increased anxiety, depression, thoughts of suicide, and interrupted breathing during sleep.

Sedatives (Barbiturates, Benzodiazepines, Z-Drugs)

Type: Highly Addictive
DEA Schedule II, III, IV Drugs
CNS Depressant

Barbiturates, Benzodiazepines, and Z-drugs all have a tranquilizing or sedative effect, which slows down the central nervous system similar to the way to alcohol works. Hostility and anxiety are common effects, along with slurred speech, and difficulty staying awake. **Sedatives can cause paranoid or suicidal ideation and impair memory, judgment, and coordination.** Tolerance and physical dependence develop with regular use, and the risk of overdose is very high with the line between a lethal dose and a safe dose being very thin.

CNS depressants and other drugs which also act as GABA agonists, are known to cause blackouts as a result of high dose use. Sedatives are some of the most commonly prescribed medications in the United States.

When people without prescriptions obtain and take these drugs for their calming and muscle relaxant effects, use turns into abuse. During times of stress, the body can become depleted of necessary neurotransmitters causing one to feel anxious and fearful. A person suffering anxiety often seeks medical attention and is ultimately prescribed these meds.

Adverse Reactions: slurred speech, staggering, poor judgment, drowsiness, reduced attention span, constant confusion, shakiness, amnesia, slowing of senses and reaction time, addiction, delirium.

Sedative Withdrawal - The first stage is minor withdrawal with anxiety, tremors, agitation, elevated systolic blood pressure, and sleeping problems. Stage two often includes auditory and visual hallucinations, heart palpitations, elevated blood pressure, and vomiting. Delirium Tremens occur in stage three of the withdrawal phase, accompanied by derealization and the inability to recognize familiar persons or objects.

Barbiturates

Amytal® (amobarbital)

A preanesthetic for surgery, but Amytal has also been controversially used as a "truth serum" in psychiatric interviews. It has been reported that a fatal dose of Amytal can be between only two to six grams, although some have died from one gram.

Phenobarbital

Primarily used as a sedative, but it is also utilized as an anticonvulsant in sub-hypnotic doses. It works by controlling the abnormal electrical activity in the brain that occurs during a seizure. This medication is also used for a *short time* to help calm or help sleep during periods of anxiety.

Seconal® (secobarbital)

Hypnotic primarily used as a sedative before a medical surgery.

Benzodiazepines

Ativan® (lorazepam)

Prescribed for anxiety, insomnia, seizures, and is also used for alcohol withdrawal. Ativan is only recommended for short-term use to avoid dependence on the drug, which can happen quickly.

Halcion® (triazolam)

Primarily prescribed for insomnia. This medication may cause daytime drowsiness. Many people experience sleepwalking episodes, and the risk increases when used with alcohol or other medications.

Klonopin® (clonazepam)

An anticonvulsant or antiepileptic drug, prescribed for panic disorders, anxiety, and to counteract undesirable side effects of antipsychotic or antidepressant medications.

Librium® (chlordiazepoxide)
A prototype often prescribed for the relief of anxiety, and to assist in the withdrawal from alcohol and other sedatives.

Restoril® (temazepam)
Tolerance to Restoril occurs very quickly, leading to harsh side effects and debilitating withdrawal effects.

Tranxene® (clorazepic acid)
Prescribed in the short-term for anxiety disorders, to prevent epileptic seizures, and to aid in alcohol withdrawal.

Valium® (diazepam)
Prescribed in the short-term for moderate anxiety, assisting in alcohol detoxification, and to prevent seizures. It also is used for presurgical sedation, and for the relief of secondary injury-related muscle spasms.

Xanax® (alprazolam)
Generally prescribed as a sedative to treat anxiety and panic disorders. It is potent and short acting and has a risk for dependence after as little as 2 weeks.

Z-drugs

Schedule Z-drugs are sedatives, but non-benzodiazepine drugs, although their effects are similar to benzodiazepines. These drugs are primarily prescribed to people with sleep problems. Sedatives are central nervous system (CNS) depressants, which slow down and decrease brain activity, resulting in feelings of drowsiness or relaxation.

Many types of sedatives have the potential for abuse, and misusing these drugs can lead to severe complications. Z-Drugs have shown to cause both physical and psychological dependence after high doses or long-term use.

Lunesta® (eszopiclone)
A sedative–hypnotic that acts on the brain to produce a calming effect to treat insomnia. It is believed that this drug interferes with deep sleep that is necessary for short-term memory to be recorded in the hippocampus and then transfered to long-term memory in the cortex. **Side Effects** are memory loss, mental/mood/behavior changes such as new or worsening depression, abnormal thoughts, thoughts of suicide, hallucinations, confusion, agitation, aggressive behavior, and anxiety.

Ambien® (zolpidem)
A powerful hypnotic sedative, depressant med that acts swiftly on the central nervous system to induce sleep by way of its "knockout" effect that induces unconsciousness. **Side Effects** can result in sleep disturbances, sleepwalking, physical discomforts, mental distress, and bizarre unpredictable reactions.

One of many reports - Ambien Induced Sleep Walking Episode:

> A mother took an accidental double dose of Ambien and it resulted in a sleepwalking event. While *sleepwalking*, she woke her two children in the middle of the night and insisted they get dressed and ready for school. Despite the children's objections, she loaded them in the car, *drove* them to school, *drove* home, and returned to bed. She awoke to her morning alarm and panicked when she realized that her children were not in their beds.

Intermezzo® (zolpidem)
A sedative or hypnotic used to treat insomnia, characterized by middle of the night waking followed by difficulty returning to sleep. **Side Effects** are confusion, depression, fast heart rate, and trouble sleeping.

Sonata® (zaleplon)
A hypnotic that alters the brain to signal relaxation and falling asleep. **Side Effects** are dizziness, drowsiness, short-term memory loss, lack of coordination, hallucinations, and thoughts of suicide.

PsychoStimulants (Amphetamines)

Type: Highly Addictive
DEA Schedule II Drugs

Stimulants are a class of psychoactive drug that increases activity in the brain. These drugs can temporarily elevate alertness, mood, and awareness. Some stimulant drugs are legal and widely used, although, many stimulants are misused and highly addictive. They are generally prescribed to combat the symptoms of ADD/ADHD, obesity or weight problems, binge-eating disorders, and sleep disorders.

Street names: Biphetamine, Addies, Bennies, Black Beauties, Crosses, Hearts, LA Turnaround, Speed, Truck Drivers, Uppers.

Side Effects: Increased heart rate, blood pressure, body temperature, and metabolism; Irritability, nervousness, feelings of exhilaration, increased energy, mental alertness, sudden outbursts of words or sounds, mood swings, tremors, reduced appetite, anxiety, panic, paranoia, violent behavior, suicidal thoughts, delirium, and psychosis. **Very serious interactions with Alcohol can occur.**

Health Risks: weight loss, insomnia, stroke, cardiac or cardiovascular complications, fainting, seizures, and addiction.

- **Adderall® (amphetamine and dextroamphetamine)**
  Widely and illegally used as an athletic performance enhancer, cognitive enhancer, and recreationally used as an aphrodisiac and euphoriant. This substance is highly potent and has a very high risk of addiction.

- **Concerta® (methylphenidate)**

- **Desoxyn® (methamphetamine)**

- **Dexedrine® (dextroamphetamine)**

- **Vyvanse® (lisdexamfetamine)**

Miscellaneous Rx Drugs

Neurontin® (gabapentin)
Released in the early 1990's, soon became one of Pfizer's most profitable drugs until litigation for misleading claims and increased suicide risk markedly dampened such enthusiasm. Neurontin is not FDA-approved for general pain relief, it is prescribed to treat epilepsy and pain related to nerve damage. "The FDA warns about **serious** breathing problems with seizure and nerve pain medicines gabapentin (Neurontin, Gralise, Horizant) and pregabalin (Lyrica, Lyrica CR) when used with CNS depressants or in patients with lung problems" (FDA.gov, 2019).

Side Effects of gabapentinoids include drowsiness, dizziness, blurry or double vision, difficulty with coordination and concentration, and swelling of the hands, legs, and feet. Withdrawal from gabapentin includes insomnia, rebound pain, and flu-like symptoms.

Serious Side Effects are an increase in suicide and violent deaths.

Belsomra® (suvorexant)
A sedative-hypnotic used for treating insomnia. The drug depresses the action of the brain's natural neurotransmitter Orexin, which is a central promoter of wakefulness. It is a federally controlled substance (C-IV) because it can be abused or cause dependence.

Side Effects: sleepiness during the day, not thinking clearly, acting strangely, confused or upset, sleepwalking or doing other activities when asleep like eating, talking, having sex, or driving a car, plus abnormal thoughts and behavior.

Some experience a more outgoing or aggressive behavior, confusion, agitation, hallucinations, worsening of depression, suicidal thoughts or actions, memory loss, anxiety, temporary inability to move or talk (sleep paralysis) for up to several minutes while going to sleep or waking up, temporary weakness in the legs that happens during the day or at night.

Part Three: Medical Madness
Neuropharmacology

Using pharmaceutical drugs to treat mental disorders is like putting an infected bandage on an open wound. Sure it will cover it up and make it look better, make everyone assume healing is taking place, but under the surface more problems are festering and the wound will most likely turn into a much bigger problem.

We have been working on developing this program for 20 years and it has come together very well. The first day of treatment produces phenomenal improvements and it keeps on working. We are finding this treatment program to be a viable alternative to Medication Assisted Treatment.

"Medical Madness – Given the momentum behind MAT, not to mention the support it enjoys among members of the nation's medical commercial and political elite, addiction may be destined to endure as one of the worlds least understood and mistreated social maladies."
- Journalist Ajay Sinijh, 2018

Thousands of people have enjoyed the benefits of our non-pharmaceutical program. It is not surprising that one may find our treatment plan incredible – because it is. During the time our patients are receiving their 2-4 hour amino acid IVs, they do not just sit in a recliner and look at the ceiling, they are a captive audience. During their daily stay, we provide group and individual therapies, such as trauma therapy, meditation, relapse prevention, massage, etc.

In fact, during the 15-20 minute Low Energy Neurofeedback (LENS) sessions, it is ideal for patients to work through a Ross Trauma Therapy curriculum. Dr. Ross has designed a model that can do more in 10 minutes than a traditional Psychiatrist typically accomplishes in a 50-minute couch session. Then, for the remainder of the day our patients may engage in Yoga, AA, acupuncture, attorney and social service visits, child visits and all the other therapies described in our treatment model.

Medical madness describes the Brain-Disabling Theory and the negative aspects of the Psychopharmacological Complex as described by the well-known psychiatrist, Dr. Peter Breggin. He notes that psychotropic treatments act by disabling normal brain functions and cause generalized brain dysfunction. They may cause typical signs of severe brain dysfunction such as euphoria, apathy, and indifference and may lead to poor judgment such as violence, suicide, and crime (Breggin, 1994-2014).

Dr. Colin Ross (2019) reports from his Trauma Model, "Throughout psychiatry, medications tend to be prescribed on a 'hit or miss' fashion, often with four to six prescribed at a time. This is too often the case regardless of the diagnosis, be it schizoaffective disorder, rapid cycling bipolar mood disorder, borderline personality disorder, schizophrenia, or other problems. The pattern has been called irrational polypharmacy, but sadly, this is the norm in psychiatry.

Psychiatrists not uncommonly make the following prescribing errors:

· Too many medications prescribed at one time.

· Dosage is too high or too low.

· Different medications are started, stopped, increased, and decreased within a short time period, often with little clarity or certainty regarding the reasons for making such change.

· Medications are not managed with clarity of diagnosis.

· Medications are prescribed for reasons not supported by scientific data (so-called off-label uses).

· Medications are prescribed for too long or too short a time period.

· Symptoms are not documented or tracked systematically.

· Medications with opposite actions are prescribed simultaneously. For instance, stimulant and a sedative may both be prescribed at one time.

· Addictive medications are prescribed to known medication abusers.

· Patients are discharged on high doses of numerous medications without adequate follow up.

· Side effects and drug–drug interactions are not recognized and/or not fully explained to patients.

- Patient noncompliance is often attributed to a bad attitude from the patient even when their prescribed medications make no sense, are not helping, or are toxic.

- Patients are told that improvement is definitely due to medications, when improvement could be due to numerous other factors.

- Patients are often told that medications are required because they have a biological illness when this theory has not been demonstrated scientifically.

- The effectiveness of medications is overstated, while the effectiveness of psychotherapy is understated.

Medical professionals have developed creative, non-medication regimes to treat the underlying causes of addiction, with an 80% sustainable recovery rate, despite receiving no addiction training during their medical school experience. Their counterparts, the prescribing physicians, (who also received no addiction training in medical school) have relied on Big Pharma for training, monetary rewards, and often on false information, resulting in an 80% relapse rate.

A brief sampling of some of the scientists who have chosen to treat the causes of addiction rather than the symptoms include: (Adkins, 2019; Blum, 1984; Cass, 2015; Glenmullen, 2000; Levine, 1997; Maté, 2009; Pert, 1997; Ross, 2007; Siegel, 2003; Van der Kolk, 1994). For a 5-decade literature review of these admirable men and women see Miller, 2019a; 2019b, as well as others mentioned in this publication.

The Future of Recovery - Further extensive research is needed to clarify the range of acute and longer-term mental, behavioral and physical effects of psychiatric drugs, both during and after consumption and withdrawal, to enable users and prescribers to benefit from their psychoactive effects judiciously, in a safe and more informed manner (Miller, 2019). The psychoactive effects of psychiatric medications have been obscured by the false presumption that these medications have disease-specific actions. More help is needed to support people who wish to discontinue psychiatric medication when it is considered safe to do so, and further research should clarify the full range of withdrawal effects and their likely duration, since there are reports of protracted and disabling withdrawal states following the discontinuation of some prescribed drugs (Precourt, et al., 2005).

General physicians and healthcare workers need more information and training about devising tapering schedules, recognizing withdrawal-related symptoms and distinguishing them from prior symptoms, in order to improve their confidence and ability to support people who wish to withdraw from prescribed medication (Cohen, 2007).

Therapy focusing on finding alternative techniques for managing emotional states, such as that provided in drug and alcohol rehabilitation programs may be necessary for people who have been on mind-, mood-, and behavior-altering drug treatment for long periods.

Approaching psychiatric medications as drugs which produce immediate and delayed psychoactive effects, and which induce tolerance and dependence, fundamentally differs from the conventional understanding that suggests these drugs exert specific actions on (presumed) underlying disease processes. According to the conventional view, the drugs' psychoactive properties are merely incidental 'side effects'.

The 5-decades of enormous literature on psychoactive effects of medications is particularly helpful, because these studies provide a baseline to which the current experimental treatments can be compared. Psychoactive effects can themselves directly modify mental and behavioral symptoms and thus affect the results of placebo-controlled trials. These effects and their impact also raise questions about the validity and importance of modern diagnosis systems. Exploiting the parallels and contrasts of conventional psychoactive medications with the psychoactive effects and uses of recreational substances helps to highlight the much broader psychoactive properties and consequences of psychiatric medications.

Some psychiatric medications produce pleasurable psychoactive effects, or even euphoria, and have consequently become drugs that some people use recreationally. Sometimes they indulge in them excessively revealing serious potential for abuse. This has been the fate of stimulants like amphetamine, introduced as a treatment for depressive neurosis in the 1940s (Rasmussen, 2006).

The misleading nature of psychiatric medications - Drugs commonly called antidepressants produce various psychoactive effects. The sedative effects of tricyclics may be useful for treatment of insomnia, anxiety, or agitation and these effects are not restricted to people with a diagnosis of depression, as reflected in the continuing popularity of low-dose tricyclic prescribing (Moncrieff, 2012).

The ability to flatten, dull or mask emotions may explain why neuroleptics are distinguished from placebo in trials of depression (Robertson & Trimble, 1982) and this, combined with their sedative effects, would also explain why many people find them helpful in anxiety (Maher, et al., 2011).

Benzodiazepines may be preferable on safety grounds, however, if temporary sedation is what is intended, because they act rapidly and their effects are generally relatively brief (4-6 hours). The benefits of other tranquilizers are not so clear. The emotional flattening or disengagement described in relation to SSRIs may reduce feelings of depression, but the generalized nature of this effect, and its frequent association with loss of libido (Goldsmith & Moncrieff, 2011) would argue against the utility of these drugs in depression.

We can speculate on how other psychoactive drugs – such as amphetamines (which induce euphoria) were long used as antidepressants, and opiates (which produce emotional anesthesia) might reduce or mask depressive symptoms. Drugs that produce short-term mood elevation or dull the emotions, however, typically require increasing doses to maintain this effect and often leave people with dysphoria when they are discontinued. Although the initial relief is recognized, often it is not long lasting and the medications can be habituating or addictive. These substances do not produce long-term mood elevation, which hints at the misleading nature of the term "antidepressant" (Moncrieff & Cohen, 2006).

> "In summary, the benzodiazepines can produce a wide variety of abnormal mental responses and hazardous behavioral abnormalities, including rebound anxiety and insomnia, psychosis, paranoia, violence, antisocial acts, depression, and suicide."
>
> – Dr. Peter Breggin

Do benefits outweigh the harm? The use of psychiatric drugs is only worthwhile if the benefits outweigh the harm. Calculating a harm/benefit ratio is a complex undertaking, however, given that what is considered harmful or beneficial varies according to many factors, such as the perspective of the observer and the phase of treatment.

Individuals will also have different subjective responses to prescribed drugs, just as people respond differently to recreational substances. The lack of data about the consequences of the long-term use of prescribed psychiatric medications on the full range of human emotions and cognitive functions further hampers a thorough and balanced assessment of their benefits or harms, especially since they are normally prescribed for months or years.

Moreover, it is often the subtle and easily overlooked aspects of drug treatment that users find most troubling. The mental effects of antipsychotics, for example, can be experienced as more unpleasant and impairing than their physical effects, and can interfere with people's ability to carry out daily tasks (Awad, 1993 & Moncrieff, et al., 2009).

The harm of psychiatric medication – It is now accepted that all major classes of psychiatric medication produce distinctive withdrawal effects, which mostly reflect their pharmacological activity. These effects are significant not only because they can prevent someone from stopping medication when they do not need it or want it anymore, but also because they may be – and probably often are – mistaken for signs of relapse (Moncrieff, 2006). This creates a situation whereby patients become psychologically as well as physically dependent on their medication, since they (and their prescribers too) may come to believe that they cannot manage without it.

Since drugs like antidepressants and antipsychotics are being prescribed for longer and longer periods suggests that some people may find it difficult, either for physical or psychological reasons, to stop medication once it is started (Moore, et al., 2009 & Prah, et al., 2012).

"The important point is that many of the approaches employed by traditional health care practitioners have serious limitations because they fail to treat the underlying causes of disease pathologies. Rather, they are largely focused on symptom suppression/elimination. Symptoms, of course, are a manifestation of the disease, but they are not the disease, and blocking them in no way addresses the cellular pathology inside the diseased cells" (Levy, 2019).

Implementing a MAT program in our prisons and jails may seem like a good idea in theory. Although, the criminal justice system will eventually adhere to their familiar punishment culture, and assume they have the power to chemically restrain any and all inmates, for any reason. Medications are only helpful in the short term, for extreme cases, and must be administered and titrated in a safe and stable environment.

Let's explore alternative strategies. When the nature of the useful effect is identified, however, other non-drug-based ways of achieving the same result may be devised that avoid the potentially harmful consequences of drug exposure (Macready, 2012). Similarly, recognizing the psychoactive effects of psychiatric medications may facilitate the development of alternative strategies for ameliorating mental distress, and also draw attention to some potentially anti-therapeutic consequences of using psychoactive substances as therapeutic agents.

Radical Change of Thinking

> "Clinical medicine inches forward at an incredibly slow rate, when it advances at all."
>
> – T. E. Levy, 2019

Despite six decades of intensive research in neuropharmacology, however, there is a lack of evidence that psychiatric drugs have a disease-specific action independent of their demonstrable psychoactive impact.

These facts suggest that a radical change of thinking may be necessary about the nature, possibilities, and limitations of psychiatric drug treatment.

Lessons from the use and misuse of other psychoactive substances can help to enlighten us about the broad range of behavioral effects that different psychiatric medications are likely to exert, and how these effects might interact with the psychological, behavioral, and other problems we call mental disorders.

Dr. Kenneth Blum and Associates (2017) caution:

> "We encourage clinicians and neuroscientists to continue to embrace the concept of "dopamine homeostasis" and search for safe, effective, validated and authentic means to achieve a lifetime of recovery, instead of reverting to anti-dopaminergic agents disrupting feed-back sequela or promoting powerful D2 agonists compromising needed balance that are doomed to fail in the war against this devastating drug epidemic."

If you want to get people off drugs,
improve reality.

- David R. Brower

Chapter 4
The Paradigm Shift

The Science-based Paradigm Shift works on the premise that it is essential to treat the causes of addiction and criminal behavior, rather than the symptoms. It is time to stop punishing the broken, to stop judging mental disorders as moral failings. People suffering the consequences from brain injuries, traumatic stress, and mental health disorders should be offered an opportunity to receive science-based therapy.

Offenders require Integrated Treatment as high rates of mental health problems are found both in offender populations and in those with substance abuse problems. Overall, the Department of Justice is the largest and least effective mental health provider in America.

Upon any arrest due to a mental health disorder, that individual is charged with a crime that remains on their record. A felony conviction forever restricts someone from obtaining employment with decent pay and valuable work. Regardless of a person having done the work to truly change, a criminal record forever labels them as ineligible for any respectable position in teaching, law enforcement, fire fighting, driving, and many more. Simply renting an apartment, holding a professional license, obtaining credit, voting, obtaining school loans, or obtaining a passport for travel are completely out of reach.

"Informed Americans no longer view addiction as a moral failing, and more and more policymakers are recognizing that punishment is an ineffective and inappropriate tool for addressing a person's drug problems — Treatment is what is needed" (Volkow, 2018).

A scientifically based neuroscience treatment protocol will also replace the concern about the addictive and negative side-effect qualities of psychotropic medication.

From MAT and Incarceration to Science-Based Integrated Care, this is a heartfelt cry for the medical and judicial systems to consider and adopt a paradigm shift.

For successful addiction treatment, it is essential to provide people with non-pharmaceutical interventions that target the underlying causes of the addiction. Physical, mental, and emotional health disorders are the underlying causes of addiction. Incarceration only exacerbates these conditions, and the provided medications are mere chemical restraints to make inmates more submissive.

Initially, an incarcerated addict may appreciate prison. After all, inmates are given meals three times a day, a place to sleep, a roof over their head, and they will always find ways to continue using the drugs they need, even in lock-up.

When paroled or released, a former inmate continues to suffer from anxiety, depression, and possible PTSD from their prolonged time spent in such a harsh environment. Unfortunately, a high percentage of parolees join the ranks of those who decide to take their own life, to end the misery, because they cannot adapt to life on the outside.

It is expected that incarcerated addicts are suffering from a nutritional deficiency, because food budgets are not considered a high priority for a convict. In addition, criminal justice officers are not trained to understand the science-based relationship between the gut and the brain. Cheap and processed foods do not contain the nutrients and essential amino acids required to heal the body and brain.

Nutrition and neurofeedback treatments are the keys needed to transform the body and the brain back to a healthy state. With a healthy and optimally functioning system, the revelations and maturity that an addict achieves in evidence-based therapies is nothing short of miraculous.

A tried and true science-based treatment protocol (biological and psychological) must be implemented in order to help these individuals find sustainable recovery.

Science-Based Treatment Plan

A Non-Pharmaceutical Model for
Anxiety, Depression, Bipolar, ADHD, PTSD, and SUD

Each of the therapies employed in this model have a profound
effect on bringing the brain to optimal functioning.

The Model
Neural-Nutritional Therapy
Coordinated Evidence–Based Healing

Clients tend to feel better at rapid rates when beginning these treatments, and it is vital to continually remind them that their mind and body are still at a very delicate stage of recovery. The healing has only just begun, it is still a process, but *now* they have a powerful opportunity to achieve a sustainable recovery.

The brain is the ultimate command center for every human function, if it is experiencing any type of trauma, then every aspect of a person's health is vulnerable to devastating side-effects. A human brain maintains 86 billion neurons, and they use electrochemical impulses to communicate with each other. A healthy brain has the ability to synchronize these impulses into a shared resonance, much like an awe-inspiring symphony.

Initial brainwave and neurotransmitter balancing is a crucial stage in this treatment protocol. We also require fuel to survive and thrive, so naturally the brain and digestive system share an intimate connection within a person.

A successful recovery depends on maintaining nutritional balance and optimizing the performance of the brain, the digestive tract, and the messages that they send back and forth.

"The intestinal microbiota evolves from birth, changing from an immature state during infancy to a more complex and diverse ecosystem in adulthood, and plays a pivotal role in both health and disease. Disequilibrium of its homeostatic state has been shown to precipitate negative consequences leading to GI, immunological, and neurological disorders" (Ross, 2017).

> When brain chemistry comes into balance, a person actually becomes more capable of responding more quickly and more deeply to all the powerful psychotherapy techniques available. This synergistic effect increases their functioning and starts the upward trajectory allowing people to blossom in ways they were never able to before.
>
> Not only is it possible to break people out of the typical downward spiral of mental illness, but by bringing together the best of all worlds of medicine, we can help people achieve a level of functioning and happiness they have never known before (Procyk, 2018).

7 Components of Care
The Transformative Journey

We provide resources for holistic support of the body, mind, and spirit on a transformative journey to recovery. We specialize in drug-free treatments.

Each of the seven components work together to ensure the greatest opportunity for lasting recovery. Our integrated approach allows us to address addiction along with life experiences with trauma, family issues, depression, anxiety, co-dependency, boundaries, and self-esteem.

We value an integrated and holistic regime that supports the entire person — body, mind, and spirit.

Comprehensive Medical Intake - We begin designing each individual recovery plan by taking a complete client history, and then conducting targeted assessments and evaluations.

Sustainable Recovery Goals:

1. **Brain Function Repair** - Low Energy Neurofeedback Therapy, amino acid therapy, and optimal nutrition help repair the brain, gut, and the balance between them.

2. **Mindful Recovery** - Sustainable recovery is a state of mind. Learning to be at peace with oneself requires practice.

3. **Behavior and Motivation** - A wide range of evidence-based therapy including Trauma Therapy, EMDR, CBT, Emotionally Focused Therapies, psychodrama, and others keeps clients engaged and interested.

4. **Spiritual / Experiential Awareness** - Spiritual and emotional guidance provide the means for the brain and mind to coalesce.

5. **Career, Financial, and Legal** - Rebuilding career skills, finding stable work, life coaching, and legal advocates provide clients tools for financial stability and a positive view of the future. Rebuilding a life in recovery takes time, patience, and planning.

6. **Family Systems & Therapy** - Addiction is a family disease. Our program teaches clients how family systems work to shape us, and how to address communication, co-dependency, and boundary setting challenges.

7. **Sustainable Lifetime Recovery** - Clients return to their lives as healthy individuals in recovery, prepared with unique knowledge and an individualized sustainable health plan. Our program stresses the need to plan. Our clients learn relapse prevention techniques along with plans for success.

LENS Therapy
Optimizing Brain Wave Resonance

It is critical that a trained and certified practitioner
provides this therapy, utilizing specifically a
Low Energy Neurofeedback System (LENS).

*Biofeedback is a commonly known exercise for an individual to practice mental techniques. We do not utilize biofeedback training in this protocol.

Low Energy Neurofeedback (LENS) is an innovative, FDA-approved, non-invasive, and cutting-edge treatment that corrects neurological pathways compromised by physical and emotional trauma. This system utilizes advanced technology and a patented process to track brainwaves in real time and relay information back to the brain in its own unique frequencies, resetting its neural-connectivity. The LENS optimizes the functioning of the brain along with the entire Central Nervous System.

LENS Therapy has helped hundreds of thousands of individuals decrease anxiety, increase and improve attention and concentration, reduce depression, increase overall energy, regulate sleep patterns, enhance creativity, and reclaim the ability to be present.

"The system works by disrupting the maladaptive patterns, or looping mechanisms, that the brain has acquired in response to acute conditions such as birth trauma, concussion resulting from a sports accident, addiction, anoxic event, etc. Low Energy Neurofeedback encourages the brain to release these inhibitive patterns, and to adapt a higher functioning neural circuitry" (Ochs, 2006).

During intake, clients complete a psychosocial history, a sensitivity evaluation, and a Central Nervous System assessment. A CNS assessment provides a scale for individual emotions, senses, clarity, energy, memory, movement, and pain. These assessments serve as the initial guidelines for the topographic LENS Brain Mapping, and important information for the medical professional supervising prescription medication titration.

LENS Therapy sessions begin by applying sensors to the client's scalp, to observe brainwave activity. We then have a computer process this activity and extract information about key brainwave frequencies. Through a patented process, we can relay this information back to the client through the sensors applied on their scalp.

LENS Therapy sessions are generally only 3-5 minutes in length, and very gentle as most people feel nothing during their sessions. The results are reduction and/or elimination of symptoms that previously interfered with the client's quality of life.

Clients continue to show measurable improvement between sessions, and most people experience long lasting relief. We all realize that life happens, and recurrent stressful situations or new trauma can slow the recovery process. In addition, some exceptions include symptoms of progressive conditions such as Parkinson's disease and Multiple sclerosis, in which the treatments need to be ongoing to sustain the improvement.

LENS Therapy has generated positive results with those who suffer from concussive injuries, TBI, anxiety, depression, PTSD, OCD, Autism Spectrum Disorders, Stroke, Asperger's Syndrome, explosiveness, ADD/ADHD, Bipolar Disorder, MS, Parkinson's, Alzheimer's, lack of motivation, seizures, headaches, migraines, substance abuse/addiction, Cerebral Palsy, and more.

Many of our clients experience total relief from previous drug/alcohol cravings, along with the elimination of ruminating negative thoughts. We have also witnessed Low Energy Neurofeedback having a strong contributing effect in managing the debilitating effects of Wernicke-Korsakoff syndrome (Miller, 2020).

"LENS is like a reset button that unlocks the brain for optimum functioning. Neuroscientists believe that the brain's defenses against stressors and trauma create neural gridlock. The Low Energy Neurofeedback System works around these blockages addressing the brain in its own electromagnetic language. LENS allows the brain to reboot, restoring optimal functioning." — David Dubin, MD

The **LENS Brain Map** creates a composite of the standard 21 EEG sites and measures the Alpha, Theta, Delta and Beta brain waves to generate a surface map and bar graph report of the amplitudes and frequencies, along with rank orders for each receptor site. The system may be utilized as a primary treatment or as an adjunct to other therapies.

In a mature brain, the ability of the DNA function is only as good as the transport system of the electrical charge. These charges are the energy source that sustains the body. Electrical currents are responsible for and maintain the individual's personality, controlling all bodily functions. A healthy brain processes a thought in roughly 1/3 of a second. Thus, speed of the electrical current determines a brain's real or functional age. When the voltage slows down, it dulls the edge of "personality," and in fact, of life. Further, healthy electrical currents are smooth, rather than emitted in bursts of surges.

Dysfunctional Delta Waves – A high Delta Wave ratio during awake time usually signals depression. The person may be lethargic, not moving and not attentive, have a low-level of arousal, little working memory, and an inability to focus and maintain attention. It is as though the brain is locked into a perpetual drowsy state.

Dysfunctional Theta Waves – The person may experience anxiety, behavioral activation and inhibition. They will likely be distracted and unfocused, have learning difficulties, memory problems, aberrant behavior, be fantasy prone with a spacey state of mind, chronic fatigue, and an inability to handle stress. These symptoms may be related to ADD, ADHD, head injuries, stroke, epilepsy, and developmental disabilities.

Dysfunctional Alpha Waves – When a person does not produce Alpha waves, or produces Alphas of insufficient power, the currents never reach the frontal lobes and tend to operate in Beta Wave mode producing varying levels of anxiety and stress. They may have a poor attention span and poor short-term memory, a loss of self-control, agitation, and will generally experience great emotional distress.

Dysfunctional Beta Waves – The person may become immobilized and overwhelmed, with an inability to focus or process information, plan things out, or accomplish math related tasks. He/she will likely experience anxiety, worry, thought rumination, low mental effort, agitation, be inhibited by motion, impulsiveness, and explosiveness.

Dysfunctional Pre-Frontal Cortex – The person may be in a fog, unable to focus or concentrate. He/she may be fearful, have difficulty with ethical or moral issues, lack empathy or social skills, and may be prone to addiction. The person may also have a difficult time completing tasks, be unmotivated and disconnected, along with inattention, poor planning or judgement, a slow reaction time, a lack of social awareness, and poor impulse control. He/she may become negative, depressed, or anxious, which could lead to a bipolar disorder.

Dysfunctional Central Cortex – He/she may have difficulty determining logical consequences of cognitive thinking, behaviors, or tasks.

Dysfunctional Temporal Cortex – The person may struggle to keep up a conversation, have an inability to recognize intricate rhythmic melodies or appreciate music, have memory lapses and forget to pay bills, forget to do common chores, or struggle to find necessary items such as keys, glasses, or other objects, which often results in aggressive or angry behaviors. These symptoms may be caused by head injuries.

Dysfunctional Occipital Cortex – The person may have difficulty with visual memories, writing, coloring, accurate reading, or other spatial activities. Traumatic memories or flashbacks are associated with the occipital lobes. He/she may suffer visual agnosia, such as an inability to perceive and draw complete objects, or an inability to see multiple objects at the same time. This person may be victim of stroke, TBI, and/or PTSD.

Dysfunctional Parietal Cortex – The person will struggle to attend to both sides of their visual field. He/she may have difficulty following directions, failure to recognize a simple tune, or remember faces, and is easily turned around or lost.

The Low Energy Neurofeedback System helps:

- **Cognition** – Problems sequencing, memory, providing and maintaining attention, concentration, clarity and organization.

- **Mood** – Anger, sadness, explosiveness.

- **Motor Skills** – Lack of grace, problems with eye-hand coordination, balance, and tremors.

- **Motivation** – Problems initiating tasks, shifting from one activity to another, and/or completing tasks.

- **Anxiety** – Problems with anxious system activity (too much uncomfortably-contained energy), persistent anxiety, restlessness, rumination, agitation, distractibility, difficulty breathing, palpitations, and sleep interruption.

- **Reactivity** – Hyper-reactivity, hypersensitivity, multiple chemical sensitivities.

- **Pain** – Brain-generated pain and vascular pain.

- **Addictions/Dependencies** – Lack of clarity about emotions, defensiveness, argumentativeness, and cynicism.

- **Fatigue** – Fatigue; or fatigue as a phenomenon secondary to the effort of trying to overcome pain.

- **LENS works extremely well with the symptoms of Traumatic Brain Injury, no matter how long ago the incident occurred. The trauma can be from a physical blow, a concussive injury, a psychological incident (PTSD), or any other incident(s) that results in a decrease in cognitive ability.**

Benzodiazepine Client: Results

Before & After LENS Therapy

EEG Brain Functions	Intake Brain Map	21 Weeks Later
Composite Amplitude	19 Sites Suppressed	20 of 21 Unsuppressed
Delta	10 Sites Suppressed	18 Sites Unsuppressed
Theta	16 Sites Suppressed	19 Sites Unsuppressed
Alpha	19 Sites Suppressed	19 Sites Unsuppressed
Lo Beta	19 Sites Suppressed	14 Sites Unsuppressed
Mean Beta	18 Sites Suppressed	12 Sites Unsuppressed
Hi Beta	19 Sites Suppressed	11 Sites Unsuppressed
Pre-Frontal (Fp1, Fpz, Fp2)	All Suppressed	All Unsuppressed
Delta	All Suppressed	All Unsuppressed
Theta	All Suppressed	Fp2 & Fpz Unsuppressed
Alpha	All Suppressed	All Unsuppressed
Lo Beta	All Suppressed	Fp1 & Fpz Unsuppressed
Mean Beta	All Suppressed	Fpz Unsuppressed
Hi Beta	All Suppressed	Fpz Unsuppressed
Central (C3, Cz, C4)	C3 & Cz Suppressed	All Suppressed
Delta	C3 & Cz Suppressed	All Unsuppressed
Theta	C3 & Cz Suppressed	C3 & C4 Unsuppressed
Alpha	All Suppressed	C4 Unsuppressed
Lo Beta	All Suppressed	All Unsuppressed
Mean Beta	C3 & Cz Suppressed	All Unsuppressed
Hi Beta	All Suppressed	All Unsuppressed
Temporal (T3, T4, T5, T6)	T3, T4, T6 Suppressed	T3, T5, T6 Unsuppressed
Delta	All Unsuppressed	All Unsuppressed
Theta	T3, T4, T6 Suppressed	All Unsuppressed
Alpha	All Suppressed	All Unsuppressed
Lo Beta	T3, T4, T5 Suppressed	T3 & T5 Unsuppressed
Mean Beta	T3, T4, T5 Suppressed	T3 & T4 Unsuppressed
Hi Beta	T3, T4, T5 Suppressed	T3 & T4 Unsuppressed
Occipital (O1, Oz, O2)	All Suppressed	All Unsuppressed
Delta	All Suppressed	All Unsuppressed
Theta	All Suppressed	All Unsuppressed
Alpha	All Suppressed	All Unsuppressed
Lo Beta	All Suppressed	O1 Unsuppressed
Mean Beta	All Suppressed	All Suppressed
Hi Beta	All Suppressed	O2 & Oz Unsuppressed
Parietal (P3, Pz, P4)	All Unsuppressed	All Unsuppressed
Delta	All Unsuppressed	All Unsuppressed
Theta	Pz Suppressed	All Unsuppressed
Alpha	Pz Suppressed	All Unsuppressed
Lo Beta	All Suppressed	P3 & Pz Unsuppressed
Mean Beta	P3 & Pz Suppressed	P3 & P4 Unsuppressed
Hi Beta	All Suppressed	All Suppressed

IV Amino Acid Therapy
Balancing Neurotransmitter Levels

It is critical that a licensed medical
professional administer IV treatments, using
the specific scientifically created solution.

*We recommend that clients have initial and periodic Neurotransmitter level evaluations performed to determine treatment needs for each individual.

Neurotransmitters Must Transmit So Brain Waves Can Wave

Neurotransmitter imbalances correlate with a wide variety of health conditions such as depression, sleep difficulties, fatigue, anxiety, and behavioral disorders. The function of neurotransmitters is to properly relay messages across the synaptic cleft, from one neuron to the next. There are more than 100 known neurotransmitters, but only 10 communicate between brain cells.

Overall, balance between the inhibitory and excitatory neurotransmitter systems is a basic concept of neurobiology, and is the cornerstone of applying neurobiology in a clinical setting. Balance insures that unimportant signals are terminated or ignored and that important signals are relayed and acted upon.

The vast majority of neurons are constantly receiving low-level stimulation by GABA, the primary inhibitory neurotransmitter. This is called tonic inhibition and requires a concise dominant signal from glutamate, the primary excitatory neurotransmitter, to be overcome and cause the neuron to reach action potential and fire.

Scientifically developed, amino acid intravenous therapy promotes healthy neurotransmissions, which in turn allows the brain waves to resonate and synchronize. Amino acid IV therapy and Low Energy Neurofeedback are the powerful team that provides sustainable recovery from anxiety, depression, PTSD, bipolar disorder, and addiction. Combining these two evidence-based therapies physically enhances and accelerates the effects of individual psychotherapies, creating a speedy and successful recovery.

During the late 1900s, Dr. Kenneth Blum initiated the concept of amino acids to achieve optimum health, without psychotropic medications (Blum, 1988, 1989).

Dr. Tamea Sisco (Addiction Diplomate), created a science-based and specialized intravenous amino acid formula, patented as an anti-craving formula. Her research indicates that amino acids do not work alone, but scientifically combined sources of essential components are also necessary for optimal results. Outlined below are the crucial elements of this science-based formula, specifically designed to create brain health and emotional wellness:

Magnesium - A deficiency of magnesium is one of the most common nutritional causes of mental health problems. Magnesium is necessary for relaxation, and a deficiency is a direct cause of anxiety and can trigger irritability (Procyk, 2018). Magnesium is essential for life as well as good health. Most patients enter the program with a magnesium deficiency.

Magnesium deficiencies have been associated with many disease states, including psychological and neurological conditions such as depression, anxiety, and insomnia.

Only magnesium can alleviate the impact of magnesium deficiency. Magnesium supplementation has been known to alleviate the neurological syndromes that are often the underlying causes of addiction. A recent publication, Magnesium Reversing Disease, provides an up-to-date explanation of the vital need for magnesium for food health. "One should never miss the opportunity to have magnesium added to an intravenous infusion" (Levy, 2019).

Vitamin C and **B Complex** vitamins are necessary to enable amino acids to cross the blood brain barrier and reach the brain. "Magnesium is the natural partner with Vitamin C in the treatment of all medical conditions" (Levy, 2019). "B vitamins are necessary to handle stress appropriately" (Procyk, 2018).

Vitamin B-12 - Vitamin B12 is simply a water-soluble vitamin that the body absolutely needs in order to ensure that nerves and blood cells stay healthy. It plays an essential role in the formation and metabolism of red blood cells, as well as in the ability to produce DNA (the genetic material in cells). B12 and Folic Acid are necessary to prevent anxiety, depression and fatigue.

Folic Acid and trace minerals are essential co-factors that drive amino acids into the cell membrane. Deficiencies of these elements can be contributing factors in many physical and psychological problems.

L-Glutamine - This amino acid supports energy metabolism in the brain, reducing symptoms of low blood sugar. It is used to reduce cravings for alcohol, sugar, and other addictive substances. It also supports liver function and has an anti-inflammatory effect on inflamed or irritated mucosal tissues.

It should be taken on an empty stomach, to avoid stomach acid, which changes its function, and degrades its effectiveness.

Glutathione - A tripeptide derived from glutamine, glycine, and cysteine amino acids. It is an antioxidant that can be synthesized in all cells of the body. Glutathione is involved in many biological processes such as free radical neutralization, detoxification, transport and storage of cysteine, maintenance of cellular redox, ascorbic acid and vitamin E regeneration, transport of mercury out of cells and brain, and serving as a coenzyme.

Glutathione is also involved in iron metabolism, including sensing and regulation of iron levels, iron trafficking, and synthesis of iron cofactors. It is believed to help maintain the integrity of the blood-brain barrier.

Glutathione is important for supporting functions of both the innate and adaptive immune systems, including T-lymphocyte proliferation, phagocytic activity of polymorphonuclear neutrophils, dendritic cell function, and antigen presentation by antigen-presenting cells.

D-Phenylalanine (DPA) - A synthetic amino acid, was created to lower the need for morphine in post-operative patients. It is well researched for its effectiveness in supporting the opioid neuropeptide: Endorphin. Endorphins relieve pain and induce feelings of pleasure and euphoria. The symptoms of endorphin depletion are generally addictions to pornography, gambling, and shopping, as well as being overly sensitive to physical pain, loneliness, and grief.

This amino acid is indicated when withdrawing from the opiate family of drugs, cannabis, and alcohol. It is available over-the-counter as DLPA, which is a combination of DPA and its mirror form L-phenylalanine, which is precursor for L-Tyrosine.

Tyrosine - An amino acid that increases energy, stress resilience, and focus by supporting the two neurotransmitters Dopamine and Norepinephrine. The symptoms of Dopamine and Norepinephrine depletion are fatigue, apathetic depression, and ADHD.

Tyrosine is indicated when withdrawing from stimulant drugs, such as caffeine, cocaine and methamphetamines, as well as, alcohol, opiates, and sometimes cannabis.

5HTP/L and Tryptophan - These amino acids reduce social anxiety, panic and phobias, agitation, obsessive thinking, and carbohydrate craving by supporting the neurotransmitter Serotonin. Serotonin is a precursor to Melatonin, which signals the brain to sleep. The symptoms of Serotonin depletion are insomnia caused by worry and rumination, anxious agitated depression, overwhelming shame, worry, irritability, sugar craving, and/or social phobia.

5HTP and Tryptophan are indicated when withdrawing from a selective serotonin re-uptake inhibitor (SSRI), cannabis, alcohol, and ecstasy.

L-Theanine - Another calming amino acid, L-Theanine is especially recommended for people with ADHD who feel overwhelmed. This amino acid has several interesting properties. It can block Glutamate, Cortisol and Norepinephrine, which may cause anxiety and agitation, and can support the neurotransmitters, dopamine, GABA, and serotonin, often leading to calm, focused attention.

It can be helpful at night for the type of insomnia caused by high cortisol at bedtime. It is sometimes identified as 'Sun-Theanine'.

Gamma Amino Butyric Acid (GABA) - An amino acid, and neurotransmitter that blocks impulses between nerve cells in the brain. Researchers suspect that GABA may boost mood or have a calming, relaxing effect on the nervous system. The symptoms of GABA depletion are muscle tension, anxiety, chronic pain, panic, seizure activity, feeling overwhelmed, being a 'highly sensitive person', and insomnia due to muscle tightness.

This amino acid is indicated when withdrawing from benzodiazepine drugs, alcohol, or cannabis.

Caution: GABA can cause anxiety and agitation in some people when used in amounts over 500mg at one time, therefore formulas where it is combined with taurine, glycine, inositol (vitamin B8), and other calming agents are recommended.

There is a recent exploration of the role of GABA in psychiatric treatment, presented by Dr. Charles F. Zorumski (2019). He states, "There's real potential in the GABA sphere for new treatments in psychiatry." He notes that we are in need of new treatments, to deal with psychiatric illness that is causing a lot of disability and death, where currently used medications are producing only fair responses with significant remission rates but with high relapse rates.

GABA is the major inhibitory neurotransmitter in the brain and is used in 20% of the synapses in the nervous system. "It is one of the main things that's available for fine-tuning neural circuits, particularly in key regions of the brain like the hippocampus." (Airov, 2019).

Nutritional Psychiatry & Exercise
Relapse Prevention Foundations

Functional Medicine Recovery

To truly help people achieve optimal functioning, and rise to the challenge of healing past and present trauma, biochemistry and physiology need optimization. LENS Therapy and IV nutrients dramatically accelerate the healing process by giving the body the raw materials it needs to function the way it is supposed to, and begins a true healing process. However, to manifest full healing, optimal functioning, prevent relapse, and maintain long-term sobriety, the physiological imbalances that led to the addiction in the first place need addressing.

"Eat real food. Our knowledge of nutrition has come full circle, back to eating food that is as close as possible to the way nature made it. Based on a solid foundation of current nutrition science, Harvard's Special Health Report (2016) Healthy Eating: A guide to the new nutrition describes how to eat for optimum health."

Digestion, inflammation, hormones, blood sugar, and neurotransmitters ALL need to be functioning properly for the body and brain to be in balance. If these issues are not comprehensively addressed, none of the other therapies will reach their full potential. Pharmaceutical interventions can be helpful to mitigate damage from these disease processes, but will never help the body actually heal.

Adjunctive Nutritional Treatments for Psychiatric Disorders

A recent meta-review by Dr. Joseph Firth of Western Sydney University in Australia states:

> "We have brought together the data from dozens and dozens of clinical trials conducted all over the world, in over 10,000 individuals treated for mental illness. This mass of data has allowed us to investigate the benefits and safety of different nutrients for mental health conditions—on a larger scale than what has ever been possible before."

Published in World Psychiatry, this review provides strong evidence for nutritional adjunctive treatments for psychiatric disorders. Dr. Firth also commented that, "The age-old saying 'healthy body, healthy mind' really is true."

Nutritional therapy is often more effective than medications in many cases. For example, research shows that a serotonin deficiency causes depression.

Dr. Anne Procyk (2018) stated:

> "The key to understanding someone's depression is understanding, why the serotonin is low, not just giving an SSRI to make the serotonin last longer. Prozac may help, but identifying why it is low is key to figuring out what the real cure is."

Another Australian study found that people who switched to a healthier diet had fewer symptoms of depression after just three weeks. Those who continued healthy eating for three months continued to feel relief from their symptoms. The lead study author, Dr. Heather Francis of Macquarie University in Sydney, Australia stated, "This has 100% reach (since everybody needs to eat), is more cost effective than medications, and is an aspect of treatment that individuals can control themselves."

You are what you eat. "Food will never be a quick fix to a crisis, but very often it is key to breaking out of the cycle of repeated crisis" (Procyk, 2018). Strategically integrated into the neurofeedback and amino acid IV components is nutrition.

Our experience shows us that self-care and proper nutrition are the keys to achieving sustainable recovery and preventing relapse. "Improving people's relationship with food and helping them learn to value food and enjoy eating in a whole new way is fundamentally about helping them learn a whole new level of self-care" (Procyk, 2018).

Proper brain function requires the presence of all essential nutrients.

The best way to get a full range of essential nutrients is to eat unprocessed foods; whole, fresh, natural foods. Another requirement for proper brain nutrition is that most carbohydrates should be complex carbohydrates from high-fiber foods, and simple sugars kept to a minimum. Derive protein from whole grains, legumes, lean meats and vegetables, and keep fats to no more than 20% of total caloric intake (Miller, 2019).

Exercise Affects The Brain

"People tend to think of exercise for weight loss or heart health, but while physical activity is necessary not only for physical health, it is also necessary for mental health. The human brain functions better when the body is physically active" (Procyk, 2018).

The human brain functions better when the body is physically active.

Physical Exercise:

- Releases endorphins that diminish pain sensations and improve sleep quality.

- Stimulates neurotrophic release to help the brain form new synaptic pathways involved with the formation of memories. Neurotrophic factors (NTFs) are a family of biomolecules – mostly peptides or small proteins – that support the growth, survival, and differentiation of both developing and mature neurons.

- Triggers hormonal changes to benefit mood and energy.

- Stimulates thyroid function, which increases metabolism to also improve mood and energy.

- Improves adrenal function which improves mood and ability to cope with stress.

Research overwhelmingly suggests that exercise works to resolve depression, anxiety, and ADHD (Procyk, 2018).

Therapeutic Technology
Alternative Therapy

Therapeutic Machines as Alternative Therapy

Photonic Stimulator: Low-Level Laser Therapy (LLLT)

We incorporate LLLT, another pain relieving alternative, into our recovery program. The Photon Stimulator light therapy is very helpful in relieving the pain and swelling.

Low-level laser therapy is the application of light (usually a low power laser) to a pathological condition to promote tissue regeneration, reduce inflammation, and relieve both acute and chronic pain. The use of low levels of visible or near-infrared (NIR) light for reducing pain, inflammation and edema, promoting healing of wounds, deeper tissues and nerves, and preventing tissue damage has been known for almost forty years, since the invention of lasers. Originally thought to be a peculiar property of soft or cold lasers, this therapeutic approach has now broadened to include photobiomodulation and photobiostimulation using non-coherent light.

The Mighty MITO

The MITO has also been found to quiet joint and sore muscle pain, including spasms and inflammation, in addition to calming the nervous system (especially when moved over the finger, toe tips, and nail beds for a few seconds).

BioMat Therapy Eases Withdrawal Symptoms

The BioMat delivers the highest vibrational resonance deeply into all body tissues. Sessions on the mat engage the curative properties of Far Infrared Rays and Negative Ions to stimulate healing and regeneration of nerves and muscle tissue layers at a molecular level.

Trauma-Focused Adjunct Therapy
Connecting Mind, Body, and Spirit
Relapse Prevention Mastery

With brain waves and neurotransmitters in balance and properly communicating, clients have the ability to learn, evaluate, process and respond to therapeutic tools. The results are simply amazing, as clients are more receptive, enthusiastic and engaged in these techniques than ever before.

In addition to sleep, proper nutrition, and exercise, there are several complementary medicine methods that can help a person avoid relapse by working to improve overall well-being.

Science-Based Alternative Therapies as Brain Repair Modalities

Research has determined that adjunct therapies such as Acupuncture, Trauma Sensitive Yoga, EMDR, Psychodrama, Meditation, Journaling, Music, Massage, Changing Behavior, Experiential Therapy, Exercise, Visualization and others work comprehensively to bring the brain to optimal functioning.

Trauma Therapy – The PTSD effects that people suffer after experiencing traumatic events cannot be relieved by drugs, alcohol, or psychotropic medication. We practice the Ross Trauma Model and trauma therapy to help a post-traumatic stress victim understand his/her trauma and dissociation (Ross, 2019). This approach provides some great strategies for coping and stabilization.

Trauma-Sensitive Yoga – Bessel Van der Kolk introduced Trauma-Sensitive Yoga at his healing center. We gradually introduce a limited number of classic postures. The emphasis is not on getting the poses "right," but on helping the participants notice which muscles are active at different times. The sequences are designed to create a rhythm between tension and relaxation – something we hope they will begin to perceive in their day-to-day lives. A major challenge in recovering from trauma remains being able to achieve a state of total relaxation and safe surrender (Van der Kolk, 1994). Yoga and exercise have beneficial effects on mood and anxiety. The practice of yoga postures associates with increased brain GABA levels.

Meditation and Yoga – Brain researchers have detected improvements in cognition and emotional well-being associated with meditation and yoga, as well as differences in how meditation and prayer affect the brains of those who believe in God and those who do not (Jarvis, 2017). People often misunderstand the practice of meditation and view it as merely a form of relaxation. Brain research, however, is beginning to produce concrete evidence that mental disciplines and meditative practice can physically change brain functioning, and preserve and enhance numerous cognitive functions. University of Montreal scientists have shown that activities like meditation have a direct impact on the brain's production of serotonin levels. Meditation "bathes" neurons with an array of feel-good chemicals, effectively melting away the stress that leads to low serotonin levels and depression.

EMDR (Eye Movement Desensitization and Reprocessing) – Developed by Dr. Francine Shapiro in 1987, as her doctoral thesis in psychology, EMDR alleviates the distress associated with traumatic memories. After successful treatment with EMDR, affective distress is relieved, negative beliefs reformulate, and physiological arousal reduces. The year 2015 was a memorable year for the world of EMDR therapists. The Annual EMDRIA Freedom to Heal Conference in Philadelphia formally introduced Neurofeedback to over 800 participants.

Now is the time of integrating specialty therapies for successful mental health and substance abuse treatment.

Psych-K (Beyond Affirmations, Will Power, and Positive Thinking) – Neuroscience reveals that at least 95% of an individual's consciousness is actually subconscious. Split-brain research created a theory of Brain Dominance, which is the Psych-K approach. Psych-K was generated by years of research and thousands of sessions with individuals and groups. It is a spiritual process with psychological benefits, and the overall purpose is to accelerate individual and global evolution by aligning subconscious beliefs with conscious wisdom from the world's great spiritual and intellectual functions.

Psychodrama – The dramatic enactment of key life events encourages the individual to activate areas of the brain otherwise not exercised. Recasting an individual's relationship with the outside world reshapes the internal world and causes measureable changes. Psychodrama is an active and creative therapeutic approach that uses guided drama and role-playing to work through problems. Developed by Dr. Jacob Moreno, psychodrama can be effective individually or in a group.

Acupuncture – As of January 1, 2019, BlueCross BlueShield (BCBS) of Tennessee stopped covering prescriptions for OxyContin, an opioid narcotic. As an alternative, BCBS replaced the drug with the traditional Chinese practice of Acupuncture. Furthermore, acupuncture treatments release endorphins into the nervous system. Considered by many to be the natural "feel good" chemical of the human body, endorphins promote feelings of health, positive thought processes, upbeat attitudes, and promote the sense of general well-being (Miller, 2019).

Emotionally Focused Therapy (EFT) – A therapy developed by Gary Craig and based on 5,000-year-old Chinese techniques. It is a powerful method formed from the discovery that emotional trauma contributes greatly to disease. Scientific studies have shown that EFT is able to rapidly reduce the emotional impact of memories and incidents that trigger emotional-like distress. Once we reduce or remove the distress, the body can often rebalance itself and accelerate healing.

Acceptance & Commitment Therapy (ACT) – Developed by Dr. Steven Hays within a coherent theoretical and philosophical framework. ACT is a unique and empirically based psychological intervention that uses acceptance and mindfulness strategies together with commitment and behavior changing strategies. Patients gain the skills to re-contextualize and accept their private events, develop greater clarity about personal values, and commit to necessary behavioral changes.

Massage – Entire body and cranial sacral massage, which is a gentle and noninvasive form that addresses the bones of the head, spinal column, and sacrum. The goal is to release compression in those areas, which alleviates the stress and pain that most patients suffer.

Experiential Therapy – Meditation and mindfulness therapy on a weekly basis, and regularly attending anonymous meetings gives clients a sense of belonging and a renewed sense of self. We also have great faith in Native American ceremonies such as the talking circle and traditional sweat lodge. The native culture recognizes White Buffalo Calf Woman as the inventor of the traditional sweat lodge. Sweats are valued for health and hygienic benefits as well as spiritual rewards. The native culture recognized the skin as the body's *third kidney*, because sweating cleanses the body of toxins and provides a regeneration of mind and body (White Bison, 2002).

Mindfulness – Known as the father of mindfulness, Dr. Jon Kabat-Zinn made meditation and mindfulness household terms, and now he gives seminars on scientific studies of the healing nature of meditation. The practice of mindfulness affects the brain in multiple ways. On a structural level, the practice of mindfulness increases activation in the left prefrontal cortex, a part of our brain connected to positive emotional states. Additionally, continually practicing mindfulness over a period of time decreases activation in the amygdala, an area of the brain implicated in our fight-or-flight and stress responses.

Gratitude – An explosion of research on the many benefits of gratitude marks the past decade. As it turns out, gratitude is not merely an emotion that feels good; it actually holds the key to a number of psychological, physical, and social benefits as well. The Psychological Benefits of Gratitude Studies show that individuals who regularly practice gratitude perform better across a number of areas, when it comes to mental and emotional health. Indeed, gratitude links to lower rates of depression, along with helping to buffer against future depressive episodes. It also decreases the rate of depression and stress, while enhancing positive mental states such as joy, optimism, and tranquility.

Native American Medicine – The emerging field of complementary integrative health care evolves from centuries of the tried-and-true healing approaches of Native American Medicine. Porter Shimer (2004), a Princeton University graduate presents a documentary of generations of Native Americans passing down information on how they actually harvested the bountiful gifts of nature to heal mind, body, and spirit.

During the late 1700's, the Seneca Tribal Leader, Handsome Lake created the *Talking Circle*, which began the first great Native American sobriety movement. "It is a native tradition to sit in a circle and talk – to share what is in your heart," John Peters (Slow Turtle), Wampanoag Tribe. The talking circle is also a listening circle, which allows one person to talk at a time, for as long as they need to talk. We gain so much by listening. Is it a coincidence that the Creator gave us one mouth and two ears? (White Bison, 2002).

Visualization – Native American shamans applied visualization as a way of seeing yourself well. One known hypnotic ceremony required the patient to visualize a hawk, or some flesh–eating creature, to enter the ailing body and devour the cause of the disease. This imagery was followed by a positive visualization of another animal spirit that would bring the gift of lasting health. This technique often worked, and today we now understand why... By scanning the brain we can extrapolate that, "what affects the brain also affects the body."

Journaling – A 2013 study found that 76% of adults who spent 20-minutes writing about their thoughts and feelings for three consecutive days, (2-weeks before a medically necessary biopsy), fully healed a mere 11 days later. Meanwhile, 58% of the control group had not recovered. Another study concluded that even 1-hour of writing about distressing, traumatic, stressful, or emotional events helped participants. These participants were also significantly less likely to get sick, as opposed to their non-journaling counterparts.

Music Therapy – During the past two decades, new brain imaging and electrical recording techniques have combined to reshape our view of music as therapy. The brain areas involved in music are also active in processing language, executive control, and motor control. Music efficiently accesses and activates these systems, and can drive complex patterns of interaction among them. Research clearly shows that through music therapy training, auditory and motor areas in the brain grow larger and interact more efficiently (Thaut & McIntosh, 2010).

Changing Destructive Behavior – One must break the cycle of addiction in order to break the cycle of self-destructive behavior (Miller, 2019). Neurotransmitter imbalance (NTI) seen in addiction is the only physio-psychological disease for which there are criminal penalties. Mental illness and alcohol or drug abuse are intermediate factors linking diet to crime. We understand that hypoglycemic people turn to alcohol to lift their blood sugar levels. The National Institute of Alcohol Abuse and Alcoholism report a high percentage of all accident, homicide, and suicide fatalities as indirectly caused by alcohol. A poor diet can drive a person to drink, so it stands a good chance of driving someone to crime as well.

The first step down the path of healing the delinquent mind is the realization that a healthy body means a healthy mind. Crimes are not committed by criminal minds or even anti-social personalities, they are committed by whole persons. Linus Pauling suggests the Orthomolecular Approach, the right molecules in the right amounts, which leads to optimal brain function. Brain function works within a set of thousands of complex chemical processes, each of which requires the presence of the proper molecules in order to work properly.

12-Step Fellowship Programs – Dr. Procyk states, "The most important place to start with all people is by building their support network." When people face criticism of new habits, or if friends, family, and co-workers are constantly tempting them back to old habits, it is nearly impossible to build new habits (Procyk, 2018).

Scientists now understand the molecular and neurobiological basis for how 12-Step programs work. They admit that addicts can find peace and sobriety through fellowship, as participants actually experience epigenetic changes of their brain. The 12-Step programs have a purposeful design, which is to support and teach the value of a higher power. During the recovery journey, relying on a higher power is essential. Addiction is larger than any individual human, and it influences all aspects of life – mental, physical, emotional, and spiritual. Healing and achieving wellness occurs when all of these elements are in alignment and balance.

Career Counseling & Life Coaching – A life coach can work with patients to help them achieve goals, overcome obstacles, and pivot or change things in their lives. Peer Assistance programs are also very helpful for finding advocates and support groups for the professional working towards obtaining licensing in his/her field.

Family Therapy – All families fall somewhere in the continuum between painful, dysfunctional family systems, and optimally functional family systems. Essentially, the healthier the family system functions, the higher a person's sense of self-worth is displayed. Similarly, the more painful the system, the more dysfunctional the family, and the lower the sense of self-worth in each family member.

Women's Therapy (The Tools For Understanding) – Internationally recognized expert in women's health, Leslie Botha created tools and information to help women learn to perceive "symptoms" as biometric feedback from their bodies about diet, lifestyle, and the state of their general emotional, and spiritual self. These symptoms are the "tell" for conditions such as hormone imbalances, depression, mental confusion, exhaustion, autoimmune disorders, allergies, and reproductive disorders.

The Life Plan – A failure to plan is a plan to fail. The Life Plan workbook is a guide for patients requiring an honest assessment of personal strengths and weaknesses, coupled with suggested strategies for achieving success and fulfillment. It asks patients to make a commitment to Self, Family, Community and most important **Sobriety**. For continued support, we recommend the use of teletherapy services.

Teletherapy Services – A 24/7 online counseling service is available for individuals in recovery, and those suffering from trauma, grief, and other mental health concerns. The Colorado Teletherapy Services model is a HIPPA compliant platform and is designed to treat issues related to PTSD, major life-changing events, depression and grief, dissociation with the anxiety (social or generated), addiction, and unsatisfactory relationships. www.ColoradoTeletherapyServices.com

Paradigm Shift
Program Design Contributors

Ochs Labs™
The Neurofeedback Experts
Low Energy Neurofeedback System (LENS)
Photonic Stimulator (LLLT)
LENS is specifically designed to restore optimal brain function. Many have been able to reduce or completely eliminate medications.

Tamea Rae Sisco, D., DADACD
Certified Addictionologist
Chiropractic Medicine
Specializing in Amino Acid Intravenous therapies for trauma, anxiety, depression and substance use dependency. She personally developed and obtained two patents for her specialized Intravenous and oral formulas.

Gottfried Kellermann, PhD
Mieke Kellermann
NeuroScience, Inc.
Premium products containing amino acids, botanicals, vitamins, and minerals exclusively to thousands of licensed healthcare providers.

Anne Procyk, ND
Naturopathic Physician
Integrative Primary Care
Third Stone Integrative Health Center
In addition to serving her busy practice, she currently teaches seminars nationwide on "Healing Chemical Imbalance Without Drugs: Integrative Medicine and Nutrition for Mental Health Disorders."

Colin Ross, MD
The Colin A. Ross Institute – For Psychological Trauma
Internationally renowned clinician, researcher, author and lecturer in the field of dissociation and trauma-related disorders. The Ross Trauma Model is a solution to the problem of comorbidity in psychiatry.

Gabor Maté, CM
Canadian Physician
Addiction Expert
"Human development through the lens of science and compassion."
Renowned speaker, best-selling author, and highly sought after for his
expertise. He has a background in family practice and a special interest
in childhood development and trauma, and in their potential lifelong
impacts on physical and mental health, including on autoimmune
disease, cancer, ADHD, addictions, and a wide range of other conditions.

Bessel van der Kolk, MD
Psychiatrist
Trauma Expert - Trauma Center
"Neuroscience research shows that the only way we can change the way
we feel is by becoming aware of our inner experience and learning to
befriend what is going on inside ourselves." He has focused on studying
treatments that stabilize physiology, increase executive functioning and
help traumatized individuals to feel fully alert to the present.

Francine Shapiro, PhD
EMDR Institute, Inc.
Originally developed Eye Movement Desensitization and Reprocessing,
a form of psychotherapy for resolving the symptoms of traumatic and
other disturbing life experiences. EMDR is so well researched that it is
now recommended as an effective treatment for trauma in the Practice
Guidelines of the American Psychiatric Association, and those of the
Departments of Defense and Veterans Affairs.

Peter A. Levine, PhD
Somatic Experiencing - Trauma Institute
Introduced the world to his pioneering approach to trauma therapy, the
Somatic Experiencing method, in Waking the Tiger and In an Unspoken
Voice. Now, with Trauma and Memory, he takes the next step in his work
as a scientist, storyteller, and master clinician.

Daniel Siegel, PhD
Mindsight Institute
A clinical professor of psychiatry at the UCLA School of Medicine and executive director of the Mindsight Institute. Dr. Siegel offers a mastery-level certificate course. This transformational course will show you how to apply the Mindsight Approach.

Candace Pert, PhD (1946 – 2013)
Neuroscientist
Pharmacologist
Discovered the opiate receptor, the cellular binding site for endorphins in the brain. The public is being misinformed about the precision of these selective serotonin-uptake inhibitors...

Kenneth Blum, PhD
Chief Scientific Advisor
Retired Professor of Pharmacology
World-renowned for his research on neurotransmitters in compulsive/addictive behaviors and genetics, also created the Amino Acid I.V. drip that works wonders for detoxing.

Eric Braverman, MD
Physician
Medical director of PATH (Place for Achieving Total Health)
"Since the majority of symptoms that cause us to seek medical attention involve a slowing of brain function or pause in that function, the best way to fix the body and prevent disease is by addressing brain chemistry."

Carl Pfeiffer, MD (1908 – 1988)
Physician
"We have found that if a drug can do the job of medical healing, a nutrient can also do the job. When we understand how a drug works, we can imitate its action with nutrients."

Progress
Leading The March

Enacted in 2008, the **Second Chance Act** (P.L. 110-199) authorizes federal grants that assist states, counties, and nonprofit organizations in developing and implementing programs to help formerly incarcerated individuals successfully reintegrate into the community after their release from correctional facilities.

Administered through the Office of Justice Programs at the U.S. Department of Justice, these programs have helped numerous counties provide reentry services such as employment assistance, substance abuse and mental health treatment, housing, family-centered programming, and mentoring to adults and juveniles returning to the community from prisons or jails.

A great congratulatory recognition goes out to Colorado's Mile High Behavioral Healthcare's Judicial Team! They were one of 12 recipients nationally to be awarded a Second Chance Act federal grant, with the goal of preventing recidivism, reducing crime, and improving public safety.

According to the U.S. Bureau of Justice Statistics, there are more than 11 million individuals admitted to jails each year, but only about 4 percent of jail admissions are resulting in prison sentences. In other words, 96% of detainees and inmates return directly to the community from jail. As formerly incarcerated individuals return to their communities, the Second Chance Act improves the coordination of reentry services and policies at the state, local, and tribal levels.

Since 2008, Second Chance Act programs have funded 600 grants to local and state governments and nonprofit organizations. More than one out of three of these awards have gone to county governments.

The First Step Act is a great start toward meaningful prison reform. The most ambitious criminal justice and prison sentencing reform in many years, the First Step Act (S 756) aims to cut recidivism and improve federal prison conditions, while also reducing mandatory sentences. Prior to its enactment, it had been several decades since Congress had made significant reforms to federal criminal justice and prison policies.

At the end of 2018, with several years in the making, President Donald Trump embraced the measure. With his support, the Senate approved the bill with a bipartisan vote of 87-12, followed by a House vote of 358-36. As a federal law, the First Step Act applies only to the 225,000 individuals in federal prisons and jails, which is only a very small fraction (about 10 percent) of all those incarcerated in the United States. The majority of people are locked up in state prisons and local jails, more than 1.9 million and counting, to whom these reforms do not apply (Richmond, 2019).

The **Prison Policy Initiative** is a criminal justice oriented American public policy think tank based in Easthampton, Massachusetts. This group is known as a go-to source for timely, actionable data about our criminal justice system. "We work to grow our movement by bringing in new supporters and making existing allies more effective. Our insightful data analyses and powerful graphics are designed to reshape tomorrow's debates around mass incarceration and over-criminalization."

The Prison Policy Initiative (2020) is known for delivering big results with a small budget, including:

- Bringing fairness to the prison and jail phone industry. Some children had to pay $1/minute for a call home from an incarcerated parent. Our research and advocacy led the Federal Communications Commission to lower the cost of calls home from prisons and jails.

- Uncovering the big picture on mass incarceration with Mass Incarceration: The Whole Pie. This report assembles data on everyone who is incarcerated or confined in different kinds of prisons, jails, and other correctional and detention facilities in the U.S. The main graphic has become the most widely-used visual in the field.

- Demonstrating that incarceration in every state — even those with relatively progressive policies — is out of line with the international community with the report and interactive graphic States of Incarceration: The Global Context.

- Protecting our democracy from the undue influence of the prison system. Our campaign against prison gerrymandering has changed how legislative districts are drawn in four states and 200+ municipalities.

- Protecting family visits from the predatory video call industry that seeks to replace traditional in-person visits with expensive video chats and grainy computer images. We've won in Massachusetts, California, Texas, Illinois, and Portland, Oregon, and we continue to fight to protect families and enact lasting change nationwide.

The **Drug Policy Alliance** envisions a just society in which the use and regulation of drugs are grounded in science, compassion, health and human rights, in which people are no longer punished for what they put into their own bodies but only for crimes committed against others, and in which the fears, prejudices and punitive prohibitions of today are no more. "Our supporters are individuals who believe the war on drugs must end. Together we work to ensure that our nation's drug policies no longer arrest, incarcerate, disenfranchise and otherwise harm millions."

Drug Policy Alliance (2020) has been at the forefront of many, perhaps most, major drug sentencing reforms over the past two decades:

- 2000 – California Passes Proposition 36
  Landmark treatment-not-incarceration law

- 2010 – Federal Fair Sentencing Act Signed Into Law
  Reduced the crack/powder sentencing disparity and repealed a mandatory minimum sentence for the first time since 1970.

- 2010 – New York Reforms the Rockefeller Drug Laws
  Eliminating mandatory minimum sentences and returning judicial discretion in many drug cases; Reforming the state's sentencing structure; Expanding drug treatment and alternatives to incarceration; Allowing resentencing of people serving sentences under the old laws.

- 2012 – California Reforms "Three Strikes Law"
  Californians passed Proposition 36, so no more Californians
  would be sentenced to life in prison for minor and nonviolent
  drug law offenses. Drug Policy Alliance Issues PAC was one of
  the primary financial contributors to the campaign.

- 2014 – California Scales Back Mass Incarceration
  Californians overwhelmingly voted in favor of Proposition 47,
  which changes six low-level, nonviolent offenses – including
  simple drug possession – from felonies to misdemeanors.

- 2014 – New Jersey Approves Bail Reform
  The new law allowed judges to deny bail to dangerous
  individuals. Now pretrial release decisions are made based
  on risk rather than resources and thousands of low-income
  individuals – many of whom are behind bars for a low-level
  drug law violation – will avoid unnecessary jail time.

- 2015-16 – California, Florida and New Mexico Pass Ground-
  breaking Asset Forfeiture Reforms
  These laws protect people suspected of drug law violations
  from unjust property seizures.

The VERA Institute of Justice works with government and civil leaders
to improve justice systems, and their "ReImagining Justice" projects are
active in more than 40 states. "We envision a society that respects the
dignity of every person and safeguards justice for everyone."

In the spotlight, **VERA's** campaign efforts affecting change are (2018):

- Atlanta City Council considers repurposing city jail after
  grassroots campaign.

- A community-led project raised more than $100,000 to pay
  bail for Muslims held pretrial.

- Pedro Hernandez held in jail for more than a year with a
  $250,000 bail is now headed to a different institution: college.

- Documentary focuses on the effects of mandatory minimum sentencing from outside the prison wall.

- Houston, Texas made 2017 news as incarcerated people sued, claiming high bail is unconstitutional and discriminatory.

- A nine-month investigation found former Jacksonville prosecutor C. Bustamante's cases resulted in black people receiving sentences nearly four times as long as white people.

- Del Pozo, a former officer in the New York City Police Department, publicly supports law enforcement officials carrying naloxone to reverse overdoses, treatment for incarcerated people, and alternatives to arrest for people with substance use disorders.

- Dayton, Ohio: From "overdose capital" to recovery model.

- To illustrate the challenges that formerly incarcerated people face as they reintegrate into their communities after release, a group of more than 40 policymakers, corrections professionals, and legal practitioners gathered in Port Orchard, Washington, for a reentry simulation exercise.

- We've partnered with government, community members, and local organizations in New Orleans, which for decades was the nation's leading jailer, to implement a series of initiatives that expanded alternatives to arrest and improved case processing. We also launched the city's first pretrial services program, to change how courts make bail decisions. With Vera's assistance, New Orleans has reduced its jail population by 80 percent since Hurricane Katrina. The city's incarceration rate is now at its lowest point since 1979.

- In October of 2019, New York City voted to close the scandal-scarred Riker's Island facility by 2026. This jail complex has nearly 10,000 beds and has become notorious for chronic abuse, neglect, and mismanagement.

About
The Authors

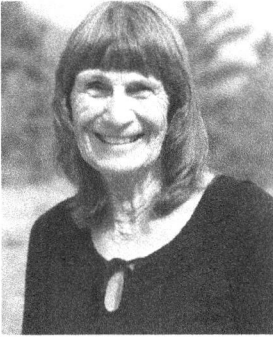

Judith Ann Miller, Ph.D., is a Colorado neuro-therapy specialist focusing on sustainable recovery of TBIs, PTSD, trauma, anxiety, depression, and substance use dependency.

She is a certified neurofeedback practitioner and employs natural nutritional regimes, and science-based psychotherapies to enhance optimal brain functioning.

Dr. Miller developed the Coordinated Alternative Therapies (CATs) model to offset the traditional, predominant Medical Assisted Therapies (MAT) model. Her premise is that it is more important to treat the causes of neural conditions rather than the symptoms.

Contact: 719-541-4912 | redfeather7@earthlink.net

Diana Eccher, M.A., is a Colorado native media design specialist with a keen interest in mental health and sustainable addiction recovery.

She embraces an idea that neuroscience, compassion, and a non-pharmaceutical approach will change the future of medicine.

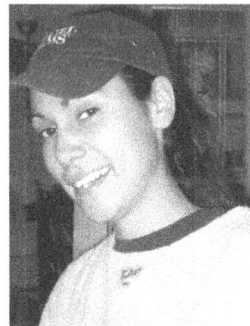

Ms. Eccher enjoys research, writing, and editing, although genuinely understanding the human condition is her focus. Her belief is that personal connection, hope, and a satisfied mind are the essential needs for moving forward in life... to be at peace.

Contact: dianaeccher@comcast.net

Glossary
Acronyms & Related Terms

The Neuro-dynamics of Broken Minds

The following is merely a partial list of terms related to the understanding of trauma related dysfunctions and are presented to give a brief understanding of the complexities. We have come a long way since, "The Three Faces of Eve."

ACE – Adverse Childhood Experiences.

ACE Inhibitors – Angiotensin-converting enzyme are heart medications that widen, or dilate, blood vessels. That increases the amount of blood the heart pumps and lowers blood pressure. They also raise blood flow, which helps to lower the heart's workload.

ACT – Acceptance Commitment Therapy.

ADA – American Disabilities Act is a civil rights law that prohibits discrimination based on disability.

ADHD – Attention-deficit/hyperactivity disorder is a neurobiological developmental disorder that can be a barrier to academic and career success. Symptoms include physical activity, inattentiveness, and impulsivity.

Alienation – Feeling unreal or cut-off from the world.

Addiction – A chronic, relapsing disease characterized by compulsive drug seeking and use, despite serious adverse consequences, and by long-lasting damages to the brain.

AFM – Affected Family Member.

Agnosia – Failure to recognize familiar objects even though the sensory mechanism is intact.

Agraphia – The inability to express thoughts in writing.

ALA – Alpha-linolenic Acid is an n-3, or omega-3, essential fatty acid.

Alexia – The inability to read.

Alexithymia – Not knowing what one is feeling, with negative thoughts of distress and depression.

Altered States of Consciousness – Characteristic deviations from the normal way people tend to perceive themselves, others, and the world around them.

Amino Acid – A molecule containing an amine group, a carbolic acid group and a chain that varies among different amino acids. Amino acids are critical to life and have many functions including the formation of proteins, enzymes, cofactors and other biochemicals.

Amnesia – Lack of memory about events occurring during a particular period of time.

Amphetamine – A psychostimulant drug known to produce increased wakefulness and focus in association with decreased fatigue and appetite. Amphetamines are believed to act by increasing synaptic activities of dopamine in the brain. i.e. Ritalin and Adderall.

Amygdala – Almond-shaped structures located deep within the medial temporal lobes of the brain that are essential for memory and Emotional reaction and are considered the limbic system.

Analytical Rumination – To think about the memory in a way that brings to mind the causes and consequences of an event.

Angry Rumination – Perseverative thinking about a personally meaningful anger-inducing event.

Anhedonia – A deficit and/or inability to experience pleasure, which is a major precursor to suicide.

Anomalous Body Experience – An out-of-body experience where the body feels as if it did not belong to itself.

Anomalous Subjective Recall – Personal memories feel if one had not been involved in them.

Anosmia – Loss of the sense of smell.

Anoxia – A condition in which there is an absence of oxygen supply to an organ's tissues although there is adequate blood flow to the tissue.

ANS – The Autonomic Nervous System, which controls heart rate, respiration, and muscle tone.

Antidepressant – A commonly prescribed psychiatric medication to alleviate mood disorders such as major depression, dysthymia, and anxiety disorders. This family of drugs includes monoamine oxidase inhibitors (MAOIs), tricyclic antidepressants (TCAs), selective serotonin reuptake inhibitors (SSRIs), and serotonin-norepinephrine reuptake inhibitors (SNRIs).

Antioxidant – A molecule capable of inhibiting the oxidation of other molecules. Antioxidants can protect the body against formation of free radicals that can damage cells.

Aphasia – Loss of the ability to express oneself and/or to understand language.

Arachnoid – Middle layer of membranes covering the brain and spinal cord.

ASD - Autism spectrum disorder is a developmental disorder that affects communication and behavior.

Asperger's Syndrome - A developmental disorder characterized by significant difficulties in social interaction and nonverbal communication, along with restricted and repetitive patterns of behavior and interests.

ASPD – Antisocial Personality Disorder is a psychiatric condition. Symptoms include stealing, narcissism, oppositional defiance, fighting, absence of remorse, and disregard for the safety of self and others.

Ataxia – Shaky and unsteady movements that result from the brain's failure to regulate the body's posture and the strength and direction of movements.

Autoscopic Hallucinations – Involves seeing one's own body at a distance or perceiving oneself as an external object, which can lead to the delusion that one has a double.

Awareness Span – Refers to things external to the self.

Axon – The nerve fiber that carries an impulse from the nerve cell to a target and also carries materials from the nerve terminals back to the nerve cell.

BBB – The blood-brain barrier consists of high intensity cells attached to blood vessels that prevent or restrict the passage of certain chemicals to the brain.

Benzodiazepines – A class of psychotropic drugs whose core chemical structure is the fusion of a benzene ring and a diazepine ring. 'Benzos' enhance the effect of the neurotransmitter GABA, which generally results in sedation, reduced activity, and improved ability to sleep.

BIAC – The Brain Injury Alliance of Colorado.

Bipolar Disorder – A serious psychiatric condition that usually involves episodes of abnormally elevated energy levels, cognition, and mood (mania) followed by episodes of clinical Depression.

Black Out – A drug-related blackout is a phenomenon caused by the intake of any substance or medication in which short-term and long-term memory creation is impaired, therefore causing a complete inability to recall the past. Blackouts are most frequently associated with GABAergic drugs.

Bp – Blood Pressure.

BPFC – Bilateral Prefrontal Cortex.

BPD – Borderline Personality Disorder people have a feeling of being overwhelmed with anger, no access to controlling their responses, or even considering the consequences of not controlling them.

Brain Stem – The stem-like part of the brain that connects to the spinal cord.

CAM – Complementary Alternative Medicine.

CATs – Coordinated Adjunctive Therapies.

CBT – Cognitive Behavioral Therapy.

Cerebellum – Brain region that has the appearance of a separate structure beneath the hemispheres. It plays an important role in motor control, the ability to have smooth physical movements, and cognitive functions such as attention and language.

Chronesthesia – Sense of time, ability to think about past or future.

CIH - Complementary Integrative Healthcare consists of products and practices not currently provided by mainstream, conventional medical practices.

Closed Head Injury – Impact to the head from an outside force, without any skull fracture or displacement.

CNS – The Central Nervous System.

Concussion – A disruption, usually temporary, of neurological function resulting from a head injury or violent shaking.

COEs – Centers of Excellence for Suicide Prevention.

Cognitive Reappraisal – Think about an event in a different, more objective and positive way.

Contusion – A bruise; an area in which blood that has leaked out of blood vessels is mixed with brain tissue.

Cortex – The cerebrum or cortex is the largest part of the brain, associated with higher brain functions such as thought and action. The Cerebral cortex is divided into four sections called lobes: frontal lobe, parietal lobe, occipital lobe and temporal lobe.

Coup & Contrecoup Injury – Brain contusions under the site of impact and on the side opposite the area that was hit; the brain bounces off the skull.

CPT – Cognitive Processing Therapy teaches one to re-frame negative thoughts about their trauma. It involves talking to a therapist about the negative thoughts and doing some writing assignments.

CSA – Childhood Sexual Abuse.

CSF – Cerebrospinal fluid is a clear fluid surrounding the brain and spinal cord.

CTE – Chronic Traumatic Encephalopathy is a progressive degenerative disease afflicting the brain of people who have suffered repeated concussions and traumatic brain injuries, such as athletes who take part in contact sports, members of the military and others.

C-TLC – Childhood Trauma Learning Collaborative.

DBT – Dialectical Behavioral Therapy.

Dehumanization – Treating people without human dignity, where the value of person is severely diminished, not only in the perpetrator's eyes, but also in victims' own eyes.

Denial – A subconscious defense mechanism used to avoid bad news. A person is faced with a fact that is too uncomfortable to accept and rejects it instead, insisting that it is not true despite what may be overwhelming evidence.

Depersonalization – Disconnected from body or watching from above.

Depressed skull fracture – A break in the bones of the head in which some bone is pushed inward, possibly pushing on or pressing into the brain.

Depression – A mental disorder characterized by a pervasive low mood, usually accompanied by low self-esteem and a loss of interest or pleasure in normally enjoyable activities.

Derealization – The feeling or perception that the world is not real.

DHA – Docosahexaenoic Acid, an omega-3 fatty acid and primary structural component in the brain, cerebral cortex, skin, and retina.

DID – Dissociative Identity Disorder. Altered States of Consciousness. Dissociation related to trauma, is the disintegration of consciousness, memory, emotion, and somatic experience.

Diplopia – A condition in which a single object appears as two objects; also called double vision.

Dissociative Catatonia – Low to no level of interaction.

DMN – Default Mode Network is one of the main intrinsic or resting-state networks in the brain, which has been suggested to play an important role in self-referential processing (SRP).

doc – Drug of Choice.

DOC – Department of Corrections.

Dopamine – A catecholamine neurotransmitter that is also a precursor of norepinephrine and adrenaline.

DPA – The Drug Policy Alliance.

DUI – Driving Under the Influence of alcohol or drugs.

Dura mater – The outermost, toughest and most fibrous of the three membranes (meninges) covering the brain and the spinal cord.

Dysarthria – Speech that is characteristically slurred, slow and difficult to understand.

Edema – Collection of fluid in the tissue causing swelling.

EMDR – Eye Movement Desensitization and Reprocessing.

Emotional Numbing – No emotions felt when weeping or laughing, unable to feel affection towards family and friends.

EPA – Eicosapentaenoic Acid, an omega-3 fatty acid.

Epidural – Located on or outside the dura mater, the outermost, toughest and most fibrous of the three membranes (meninges) covering the brain.

FEAR – False Assumption that Everything is Real.

Flashbacks – Episodic autobiographical memory recall.

FNNR – Foundation for Neurofeedback & Neuromodulation Research.

GABA – Gamma-aminobutyric acid is the chief inhibitory (calming) neurotransmitter in the central nervous system.

GERD – Gastroesophageal Reflux Disease, or chronic heartburn.

HALT – Hungry, Angry, Lonely, Tired.

Hallucination – A mistaken perception of visual, auditory, tactile, olfactory, or other sensory experience without an external stimulus and with a compelling sense of it is reality, usually resulting from a mental disorder or as a response to a drug.

Hemianopsia – Loss of part of one's visual field in one or both eyes.

Hemiparesis – Weakness, paralysis, loss of movement on one side of the body.

Hemiplegia – Paralysis of one side of the body as a result of injury to neurons carrying signals to muscles from the motor areas of the brain or spinal cord.

Hippocampus – A brain structure under the medial temporal lobe, one on each side of the brain. It is critical for the formation of new memories and has an important role in learning and behavior.

Hydrocephalus – A condition in which excess CSF builds up within the ventricles (fluid-containing cavities) of the brain and may cause increased pressure within the head.

Hyperactivity – A physical state in which a person is abnormally and easily excitable or exuberant often resulting in strong emotional reactions, impulsive behavior, and a short attention span.

Hypoxia – A condition in which there is a decrease of oxygen to the tissue despite adequate blood flow to the tissue.

IBS – Irritable Bowel Syndrome.

Interpersonal Psychotherapy – Focuses on the impact of trauma on interpersonal relationships.

Intervention – An event that presents reality (specific information) in a renewal form (with concern and compassion) to a person unable to see that reality (in denial). Often implemented to bring an addicted person to treatment.

Ischemia – A reduction of blood flow that is thought to be a major cause of secondary injury to the brain or spinal cord after trauma

Level of Arousal Activation – The ability to interact with the physical and social environment.

Loss of Self-Awareness – A dissociative person not recognizing him/herself in the mirror.

MHTTC – The Mental Health Technology Transfer Center Network, funded by SAMHSA.

MI – Motivational Interviewing is a counseling method that helps people resolve ambivalent feelings and insecurities to find the internal motivation they need to change their behavior.

MIRECC – The Mental Illness Research Education and Clinical Center to promote collaboration with VA Centers and VA Healthcare Centers for suicide prevention.

MORE Act – Marijuana Opportunity Reinvestment and Encouragement Act, which would de-schedule marijuana at the federal level, let states set their own policies without interference, and begin repairing the extensive damage done by prohibition.

MPFC – Medial Prefrontal Cortex.

MST – Military Sexual Trauma.

NABH – The National Association of Behavioral Healthcare.

NAMI – The National Alliance for Mentally Ill.

NAS – Neonatal Abstinence Syndrome.

NCPTSD – The National Center for Post-Traumatic Stress Disorder.

Neuron – An electrically excitable nerve cell that processes and transmits information by electrical and chemical signaling to other neurons across a synapse. Neurons interact with each other to form networks and are the core components of the brain and peripheral nervous system.

Neurotransmitter – A chemical that is released from a nerve cell (neuron) and transmits an impulse to another nerve cell. A neurotransmitter is a messenger of neurologic information from one cell to another. 100+ neurotransmitters are identified, including monoamines, amino acids, peptides, and other chemicals such as acetylcholine, zinc, and nitric acid.

NMS – Neuroleptic Malignant Syndrome.

NSAID – Nonsteroidal Anti-inflammatory Drug.

NSDUH - The National Survey on Drug Use and Health provides up-to-date information on tobacco, alcohol, and drug use, mental health and other health-related issues in the United States.

NWC – Normal Waking Consciousness.

OCD – Obsessive-compulsive Disorder is a mental disorder characterized by the presence of recurrent ideas and fantasies (obsessions), repetitive impulses or actions (compulsions) and high activity.

ONDCP – The Office of National Drug Control Policy Center created by the American Drug Abuse Act of 1988.

Open head injury – Trauma to the brain resulting in loss of consciousness due to the penetration of the brain by a foreign object, such as a bullet.

Opioid – A compound or drug that binds to receptors in the brain involved in the control of pain and other functions (e.g., morphine, heroin, hydrocodone, oxycodone).

PACC – Perigenual Anterior Cingulate Cortex.

Paranoia – A psychological disorder, delusions or perceptions of grandeur.

PCT – Present-Centered Therapy focuses on current PTSD problems.

Perspective (1st Person) – An experiential basis for accurate self.

Perspective (2nd Person) – Experiencing thoughts as the voices of others within one's head.

Perspective (3rd Person) – Decentered and disowned bodily experience.

Physical Dependence – An adaptive physiological state that occurs with regular drug use and results in a withdrawal syndrome when the drug is stopped; often occurs with tolerance. Physical dependence can happen with chronic – even appropriate – use of many medications, and by itself does not constitute addiction.

Polydrug Abuse – The abuse of two or more drugs at the same time, such as CNS depressants and alcohol.

PPIs – Photon Pump Inhibitors.

Prescription Drug Abuse – The use of a medication without a prescription; in a way other than as prescribed; or for the experience of feeling elicited. This term is used interchangeably with "nonmedical" use.

Protein – A large molecule composed of one or more chains of amino acids in a specific order determined by the DNA coding for the protein. Proteins are required for of the structure function, and regulation of the body cells, tissues and organs.

Psychotherapeutics – Drugs that have an effect on the function of the brain and that often are used to treat psychiatric/neurologic disorders; includes opioids, CNS depressants, and stimulants.

Psychosis – A symptom or feature of mental illness, usually characterized by radical changes in personality, impaired cognitive functioning, and a distorted sense of objective reality (hallucinations, delusions, paranoia, etc.)

PTSD – Post-Traumatic Stress Disorder.

PTSD Dissociative Subtype: Depersonalization – (often used interchangeably with out-of-body experiences) Feeling as an outside observer of the happenings of one's own mind or body – exemplified by perceptual alterations, altered sense of time, emotional or physical numbing or alterations in sense of self.

QT Interval Prolongation – A heart rhythm disorder that can potentially cause fast, chaotic heartbeats. Long QT syndrome can be inherited or caused by a medication or condition. It often goes undiagnosed or is misdiagnosed as a seizure disorder, such as epilepsy.

Respiratory Depression – Slowing of respiration (breathing) that results in the reduced availability of oxygen to vital organs.

SAD – Seasonal Affective Disorder.

SAD – Social Anxiety Disorder.

SBIRT - Screening, Brief Intervention, and Referral to Treatment is an evidence-based early intervention practice to identify, reduce, and prevent the misuse of alcohol, medications, and illicit drugs.

SAMHSA – The Substance Abuse and Mental Health Services Administration.

Schizophrenia – Psychotic disorders that commonly involve auditory hallucinations, paranoid or bizarre delusions, disorganized speech, anxiety, depression, and other symptoms that usually result in significant social and occupational dysfunction.

Sedatives – Drugs that suppress anxiety and promote sleep; the NSDUH classification includes benzodiazepines, barbiturates, and other types of CNS depressants.

Sensory Dynamics – Subjectively perceived intensity of physical sensations such as brightness of colors or loudness of sounds.

Serotonin (5–HTP) – A monoamine neurotransmitter (5–Hydroxytryptamine) biochemically derived from tryptophan that has an important role in depression and other mental disorders.

SIT - Stress Inoculation Training is a cognitive–behavioral therapy and teaches skills and techniques to manage stress and reduce anxiety.

SMITREC – Serious Mental Illness Treatment Research and Education Center.

SNRIs – Selective Norepinephrine Reuptake Inhibitors.

SOBER – Son of a Bitch Everything's Real.

SRP – Self Referential Processing entails first person perspective of, "This is happening to me."

SSRIs – Selective serotonin reuptake inhibitors are one of a family of antidepressant medications that inhibit the removal of serotonin from synapses by transport proteins.

Stimulants – A class of drugs that enhances the activity of monoamines (such as dopamine) in the brain, increasing arousal, heart rate, blood pressure, and respiration, and decreasing appetite; includes some medications used to treat attention–deficit hyperactivity disorder (e.g., methylphenidate and amphetamines), as well as cocaine and methamphetamine.

Subarachnoid hemorrhage – Blood in, or bleeding into, the space under the arachnoid membrane, most commonly from trauma or from rupture of an aneurysm.

Subdural – The area beneath the dura covering the brain and spinal cord.

Substance Abuse – When alcohol or drug use adversely affects the health of the user or when the use of a substance imposes social and personal costs. Waking the next day with a hangover.

Substance Dependence – Also referred to as addiction, is a compulsive craving for a substance. It is a chronic and progressive disease, and withdrawal is usually characterized by physiological symptoms. People who are addicted cannot function normally without the substance because their body depends on it, either physically or psychologically.

Substance Misuse – The use of a substance for a purpose not consistent with legal or medical guidelines. This term describes the use of a prescription drug in a way that varies from the medical direction such as taking more than the prescribed amount of a drug or using someone else's prescribed drug for medical or recreational use.

Substance Use – The consumption of low and/or infrequent doses of alcohol and other drugs such that damaging consequences may be rare or minor. Substance use might include an occasional glass of wine or beer with dinner, or the legal use of prescription medication as directed by a doctor to relieve pain or to treat a behavioral health disorder.

SUD – Substance Use Disorder.

TBI – Traumatic Brain Injury.

Tolerance – A condition in which higher doses of a drug are required to produce the same effect achieved during the initial use; often associated with physical dependence.

Tranquilizers – Drugs prescribed to produce sleep or reduce anxiety; the NSDUH classification includes benzodiazepines and other types of CNS depressants.

VERA Institute of Justice – The Vera Institute of Justice, founded in 1961, is an independent nonprofit national research and policy organization in the United States. Vera works closely with government to build and improve justice systems that ensure fairness, promote safety, and strengthen communities.

WHO – The World Health Organization, United Nations Group.

Withdrawal – Symptoms that occur after chronic use of a drug is reduced abruptly or stopped.

Assessment Tools
Measuring the Effects of Trauma

AUDIT – Alcohol Use Disorders Identification Test, an anonymous assessment from WHO, Department of Mental Health and Substance Dependence.

CADSS – Clinician Administered Dissociative Status Scales is a survey of acute dissociative experiences. (e.g. "Do things seem to be moving in slow motion?").

CAPS – Clinician-Administered PTSD Scale.

Centrality of Events Scale – Measures traumatized persons who consider memories of traumatic events to be central components of their personal identity.

DES – The Dissociative Experiences Scale measures a wide variety of types of dissociation, including both problematic dissociative experiences, and normal dissociative experiences (day-dreaming).

DSM-IV – Diagnostic and Statistical Manual for Psychiatric Disorders.

DSM-5 – The Diagnostic and Statistical Manual of Mental Disorders, Fifth Edition is the 2013 update, the taxonomic and diagnostic tool published by the American Psychiatric Association.

THS - The Trait Hope Scale measures a person's experience of hope. The scale measures a global experience of hope and is divided into two subscales.

Trauma Recovery Group – Group therapy to help decrease survivors' sense of social isolation can promote mastery and empowerment and can serve as a basis for the modeling of healthy relationships.

TRASC – Trauma Related Altered States of Consciousness. Designed to track 1) flashbacks of trauma memories, 2) voice-hearing, 3) depersonalization, and 4) marked-emotional numbing and affective shut-down.

MDI – Multiscale Dissociation Inventory is a 30-item self-report test of dissociative symptomatology. It is fully standardized and measures six different type of dissociative response.

MID – Multidimensional Inventory of Dissociation is a multiscale instrument that comprehensively assesses the phenomenological domain of pathological dissociation and diagnoses the dissociative disorders.

PDEQ – Peritraumatic Dissociative Experiences Questionnaire is a 10-item test that measures the extent of dissociation at the time of the traumatic event, and in the minutes and hours that followed.

PTCI – Post Traumatic Cognitions Inventory – Differentiates the content of conscious thought of traumatized people with versus without PTSD.

RSDI – Response to Script-Driven Imagery Scale – Differentiates the depersonalization (dissociative) response from that of experiencing and avoidance by phenomenological self-report in the context of trauma reminders. The RSDI is predictive of differential neural responses to trauma script-driven imagery.

SDQ-20 – Somatoform Dissociation Questionnaire – A self-report measure of Somatoform Dissociation and includes terms that overlap with depersonalization.

TAS-20 - Toronto Alexithymia Questionnaire is an instrument that measures the degree of alexithymia. People who have trouble identifying and describing emotions and who tend to minimize emotional experience and focus attention externally.

VV-SORP-T – Visual-Verbal Self-Other Referential Processing Task is a neuroimaging (fMRI) study.

References
Paradigm Shift Resources

Treating TBI, PTSD, Trauma, Anxiety, Depression, & SUD

Five decades of science-based literature are presented to
serve as supporting evidence for the fields of TBI, PTSD,
Trauma, Anxiety, Depression, and SUD, as well as supporting
evidence for decriminalizing substance use disorder, and
the misuse of MAT (Medication Assisted Therapy).

Music References

Cash, J. (1969). *San Quentin.* [Recorded Live at San Quentin State Prison, CA]. On At San Quentin. New York, NY: Columbia Records.

Hewson, P. D. (Bono). (1987). *Running to stand still.* [Recorded by U2]. On The Joshua Tree. New York, NY: Island Records.

Marley, B. (1980). *Redemption song.* [Recorded by Bob Marley and The Wailers]. On Uprising. Kingston, Jamaica: Tuff Gong/Island Records.

References

Adams, M. (2013, April 2). Every mass shooting over last 20 years has one thing in common... and it's not guns. *Natural News.* https://www.naturalnews.com/039752_mass_shootings_psychiatric_drugs_antidepressants.html

Airov, T. (2019). A real chill pill: The power of mindfulness in the treatment of anxiety disorders. Presented at *Psych Congress*: San Diego, CA.

Albright, C. (2010). *Neurofeedback: Transforming your life with brain biofeedback.* (n.p.): Beckworth Publications.

Albright, C. (2010, January 16). Neurofeedback in the treatment of addiction. *Ezine Articles.* Retrieved from: https://ezinearticles.com/?Neurofeedback-in-the-Treatment-of-Addiction&id=3589779

Alexander, B. K., Beyerstein, B. L., Hadaway, B. F., & Coombs, R. B. (1981). Effect of early and later colony housing on oral ingestion of morphine in rats. *Pharmacol Biochem Behav, 15,* 571-576. doi:10.1016/0091-3057(81)90211-2

Alexander, M. (2020). *The new Jim Crow: Mass incarceration in the age of colorblindness.* New York, NY: The New Press.

Alper, K. R., Prichep, L. S., Kowalek, S., Rosenthal, M. S., & John, E. (1998). Persistent QEEG abnormality in crack cocaine users at 6 months of drug abstinence. *Neuropsychopharmacology, 19*(1), 1-9.

Amaker, R. J., Woods, Y., & Gerardi, S. M. (2009). AOTA's societal statement on combat-related posttraumatic stress. *American Journal of Occupational Therapy, 63,* 469-470.

Amen, D. G. (2000). *Change your brain: Change your life.* New York, NY: Three Rivers Press.

Amen, D. G. (2008). *Magnificent mind at any age: Treat anxiety, depression, memory problems, ADD, and insomnia.* New York, NY: Random House.

Amen, D. G., & Routh, L.C. (2003). *Healing anxiety and depression.* New York, NY: Putnam Publishing Group.

Amen, D. G., Newberg, A., Thatcher, R., Jin, Y., Wu, J., Keator, D., & Willeumier, K. (2011). Impact of playing professional football on long-term brain function. *Journal of Neuropsychiatry & Clinical Neurosciences, 23*, 98-106.

American Psychiatric Association (2000). *Diagnostic and statistical manual of mental disorders* (4th ed., Text Revision). Washington, DC: Author.

American Psychiatric Association. (2013). *Diagnostic and statistical manual of mental disorders* (5th ed.). Arlington, VA: Author.

Anderson, F. (2016). Responding to extreme trauma symptoms: How neuroscience can help. *Psychotherapy Networker.* November/December, 2016.

Anderson, F. G., Sweezy, M., & Schwartz, R. C. (2017). *Internal family systems: Skills training manual trauma-informed treatment for anxiety, depression, PTSD, & substance abuse.* Eau Claire, WI: PESI Publishing.

Antonuccio, D. O., Danton, W. G., & DeNelsky, G. Y. (1995). Psychotherapy versus medication for depression: Challenging the conventional wisdom. *Professional Psychology: Research and Practice, 26*(6), 574-585.

Arani, F. D., Rostami, R., & Nostrabadi, M. (2010). Effectiveness of neurofeedback training as a treatment for opioid-dependent patients. *Clinical EEG and Neuroscience, 41*(3), 170-177.

Armour, J. (2010). *The body's role in addictions.* Bloomington, TN: Balboa Press.

Arnold, C. (2013) Gut feelings: The future of psychiatry may be inside your stomach. *The Verge.* Retrieved from http://www.theverge.com/2013/8/21/4595712/gut-feelings-the-future-of-psychiatry-may-be-inside-your-stomach

Arts, N., Walycort, S., & Kessels, R. (2017). Korsakoff's syndrome: A critical review. *Neuropsychiatric Disease and Treatment, 13*, 2875-2890.

Atkins, C. (2014). *Co-occurring disorders: Integrated assessment and treatment of substance use and mental disorders.* Eau Claire, WI: PESI Publishing.

Atkins, C. (2018). *Opioid use disorder: A holistic guide to assessment, treatment, and recovery.* Eau Claire, WI: PESI Publishing.

Avey, J. B. (2014). The left side of psychological capital: New evidence on the antecedents of PsyCap. *Journal of Leadership & Organizational Studies, 21*(2), 141–149. https://doi.org/10.1177/1548051813515516

Awad, A. G. (1993). Subjective response to neuroleptics in schizophrenia, *Schizophrenia Bulletin, 19*(3), 509-518. https://doi.org/10.1093/schbul/19.3.609

Ayers, M. E. (1987). Electroencephalographic neurofeedback and closed head injury of 250 individuals. Washington, DC: National Head Injury Foundation Syllabus, *Head Injury Frontiers,* 380-392.

Ayers, M. E. (1999). Assessing and training open head trauma, coma, and stroke using real-time digital EEG neurofeedback. In J. R. Evans & A. Abarbanel (Eds.), *Introduction of Quantitative EEG and neurofeedback* (pp. 203-222). Academic: New York, NY.

Bachhuber, A., et al. (2016). Increasing benzodiazepine prescriptions and overdose mortality in the United States, 1996–2013. *Am Journal of Public Health, 106*.

Bagby, R. M., & Taylor, G. J. (1994). The twenty-item Toronto Alexithymia Scale: 1. Item selection and cross-validation of the factor structure. *Journal of Psychosomatic Research, 38*(1), 23-32. doi:19.1016/0022-3999(94)90005-1

Baler, R.D., & Volkow, N. D. (2006). Drug addiction: The neurobiology of disrupted self-control. *Trends Mol Med, 12*(12), 559–566.

Barinaga, M. (2000, February 11). A new clue on how alcohol damages brains. *Science*, 947-948.

Bascarino, J., Rukstalis, M., Hoffman, S., et al. (2010). Risk factors for drug dependence among out-patients on opioid therapy in a large US health-care-system. *Addiction, 105*, 332-339.

Bauer, L. O. (2001). Predicting relapse to alcohol and drug abuse via quantitative electroencephalography. *Neuropsychopharmacology, 25*, 332-340.

Baughman, Jr., F. A. (2015, May 1-3). Soldiers of the Iraq/Afghanistan era dead of sudden cardiac death probably due to prescription antipsychotic & other psychotropic drugs. 22nd Annual *Combat Stress Conference*: Carlsbad, CA.

Baumel, S. (1995). *Dealing with depression naturally*. New Canaan, CT: Keats Pub.

Bazzi, A., & Saiz, R. (2018). Screening for unhealthy alcohol use. Journal of the *American Medical Association, 320*(18), 1869-1871. doi:10.1001/jama.2018.16069

Bearden, T. S., Cassisi, J. E., & Pineda, M. (2003). Neurofeedback training for a patient with thalamic and cortical infarctions. *Applied Psychophysiology & Biofeedback, 28*, 241-253.

Beasley, J. D. (1992). *Diagnosing and managing chemical dependency*. Amityville, NY: Professional Communications.

Beasley, J. D., & Swift, J. J. (1980). Dietary intake of certain amino acids linked to Brain Function. *Clinical Psychiatry, 8*(10), 1-20.

Bell J. (2014). Pharmacological maintenance treatments of opiate addiction. British *Journal of Clinical Pharmacology, 77*, 253-263.

Bernstein, E. M., & Putnam, F. W. (1986, December). Development, reliability, and validity of a dissociation scale. Dissociative Experiences Scale (DES). *Journal of Nervous and Mental Disease, 174*(12), 727-35.

Berntsen, D., & Rubin, D. C. (2006). Emotion and vantage point in autobiographical memory. *Cognitive Psychology, 21*(4), 417-431. doi:10.1080/02699930500371190

Binswanger, A., et al. (2013). Mortality after prison release: Opioid overdose and their causes of death, risk factors, and time trends from 1999 to 2009. *Annals of Internal Medicine, 159*(9), 592-600.

Bisaga, A., & Chernyaev, K. (2018). *Overcoming opioid addiction: The authoritative medical guide for patients, families, doctors, and therapists.* New York, NY: Experiment Publishing.

Blum, K. (1984). *Handbook of abusable drugs.* New York, NY: Gardner Press, Inc.

Blum, K. (1989). A commentary on neurotransmitter restoration as a common mode of treatment for alcohol, cocaine, and opiate abuse. *Integrative Psychiatry, 6,* 199-204.

Blum, K., Braverman, E. R., Holder, J. M., Lubar, J. F., Monastra, V. J., Miller, D., Lubar, et all. (2000). Reward deficiency syndrome: A biogenetic model for the diagnosis and treatment of impulsive, addictive and compulsive disorders. *Journal of Psychoactive Drugs, 32.*

Blum, K., Cull, J. G., Braveman, E. R., & Cummings, D. E. (1996). Reward deficiency syndrome. *American Scientist, 84*(2), 132-145.

Blum, K., Downs, W., Siwicki, D., Giordano, J., McLaughlin, T., & Neary, J. (2017, November 7). Dopamine homeostasis requires balanced poly-pharmacy: We caution against the risk-laden use of destructive powerful dopamine agents to combat America's drug epidemic. *The Sober World.*

Blum, K., & Payne, J. E. (1991). *Alcohol and the addictive brain.* New York, NY: The Free Press.

Blum, K., Siwicki, D., & Jones, J. (2018, July 1). Genetic selfie: A real time snapshot of your addictive self. *Sober World.* Retrieved from https://www.thesoberworld. com/2018/07/01/genetic-selfie-real-time-hd-snapshot-addictive-self/

Blum, K., & Trachtenberg, M. C. (1988). *Some things you should know about alcoholism.* Houston, TX: Matrix Technologies, Inc.

Blum, K., Trachtenberg, M. C., & Ramsay, J. C. (1988). Improvement of inpatient treatment of the alcoholic as a function of neurotransmitter restoration: A pilot study. *The International Journal of the Addictions, 23*(9), 991-998.

Bongiorno, P. (2012). *How come they're happy and I'm not: The compete natural program for healing depression for good.* San Francisco, CA: Conari Press.

Bongiorno, P. (2015). *Put anxiety behind you: The complete drug-free program.* San Francisco, CA: Conari Press.

Bongiorno, P. (2015). *Holistic solutions for anxiety & depression in therapy: Combining natural remedies with conventional care.* New York, NY: W.W. Norton & Company.

Boston University. (2019). Seasonal affective disorder impacts 10 million Americans. Are you one of them? *Neuroscience News.* Retrieved from https://neurosciencenews.com/seasonal-affective-disorder-1515/

Bounias, M., Laibow, R. E., Bonaly, A., & Stubblebine, A. N. (2001). EEG-Neurofeedback treatment of patients with brain injury: Part 1: Typological classification of clinical syndromes. *Journal of Neurotherapy, 5*(4), 23-44.

Bounias, M., Laibow, R. E., Bonaly, A., & Stubblebine, A. N. (2002). EEG-neurofeedback treatment of patients with brain injury Part 4: Duration of treatments as a function of both the initial load of clinical symptoms and the rate of rehabilitation. *Journal of Neurotherapy, 6*(1), 28-38.

Boynton, T. (2001). Applied research using alpha/theta training for enhancing creativity and well-being. *Journal of Neurotherapy, 5*(1), 5-18.

Bracciano, A. G. (2008). *Physical agent modalities: Theory and application for the occupational therapist* (2nd ed.). Thorofare, NJ: Slack Incorporated.

Bracciano, A. G., Chang, W. P., Kokesh, S. (2012). Cranial electrotherapy stimulation in the treatment of posttraumatic stress disorder: A pilot study of two military veterans. *Journal of Neurotherapy, 16*(1), 60-69.

Bradford, B., & Nandi, A. (2018). *Motivational interviewing in corrections: A comprehensive guide to implementing MI in corrections.* National Institute of Corrections, U. S Department of Justice.

Brady, K. T., Killeen, T. K., Brewerton, T., & Lucerini, S. (2000). Comorbidity of psychiatric disorders and posttraumatic stress disorder. *J of Clinical Psychiatry.*

Braverman, E. R., Blum, K., & Smayda, R. J. (1990). A commentary on brain mapping in 60 substance abusers: Can the potential for drug abuse be predicted and prevented by treatment? *Current Therapeutic Research, 48*(4), 569-585.

Braverman, E. R., Pfeiffer, C., Blum, K., & Smayda, R. (2003). *The healing nutrients within: How to use amino acids to achieve optimum health and fight cancer, Alzheimer's disease, depression, heart disease, and more.* North Bergen, NH: Basic Health Publications.

Bray, R. M., et al. (2010). Substance use and mental health trends among U.S. military active duty personnel: Key findings from the 2008 DoD health behavior survey. *Military Medicine, 175*(6), 390. https://doi.org/10.7205/MILMED-D-09-00132

Breggin, P. (1994). *Toxic psychiatry.* New York, NY: St. Martin's Press.

Breggin, P. R. (2007). *Brain disabling treatment in psychiatry: Drugs, electroshock and the psychopharmacological complex*. New York, NY: Springer Publishing.

Breggin, P. R. (2009). *Medical madness: The role of psychiatric drugs in cases of violence, suicide & crime*. New York, NY: Springer Publishing Co.

Breggin, P. R., & Ross, G. (1994). *Talking back to Prozac*. New York, NY: St. Martin's.

Bremmer, J. D. (1999). Does stress change the brain? *Biological Psychiatry, 45*, 797-805.

Breslau, N., Davis, G. C., Andreski, P., & Peterson, E. (1991). Traumatic events and posttraumatic stress disorder of an urban population of young adults. *Archives of General Psychiatry, 48*(3), 216-222.

Briere, J. (2002). *Multiscale Dissociation Inventory* (MID). Lutz, FL: Psychological Assessment Resources.

Britt, J. P., & Bonci, A. (2013). Optogenetic interrogations of the neural circuits underlying addiction. *Current Opinion in Neurobiology, 23*, 539-545.

Brookshire, B. (2015, January 14). To beat sleepiness of anxiety drugs, team looks to body's clock. *Science News*. Retrieved from https://www.sciencenews.org/blog/scicurious/beat-sleepiness-anxiety-drugs-team-looks-bodys-clock

Brown, A. D. (2019, October 31). Living beyond – The brain, addiction and discrimination. *The Sober World*. Retrieved from https://www.thesoberworld.com/2019/10/31/living-beyond-the-brain-addiction-and-discrimination

Brown, A. M. (2012). Acquired brain injury: A case study. *NeuroConnections*, Summer, 37-38.

Brown, P. J., Rucepero, P. R., & Stout, R. (1995). PTSD substance abuse comorbidity and treatment visualization. *Addictive Behaviors, 20*(2), 251-254.

Brown, R. J., Blum, K., & Trachtenberg, M. C. (1990). Neurodynamics of relapse prevention: A neuronutrient approach to outpatient DUI offenders. *Journal of Psychoactive Drugs, 22*(2), 173-187.

Brown, R. P., & Gerbarg, P. L. (2012). *The healing power of the breath: Simple techniques to reduce stress and anxiety, enhance concentration, and balance your emotions*. Boston, MA: Shambhala.

Bruijnen, C., Dijkstra, B., Walvoort, S., Markus, W., VanDerNagel, J., Kessels, R., & DE Jong, C. (2019). Prevalence of cognitive impairment in patients with substance use disorder. *Drug and Alcohol Review, 38*(4), 435-442. doi:10.1111/dar.12922

Bureau of Prisons. (2016). *Annual Determination of Average Cost of Incarceration*. US Department of Justice, 81, p. 46957, document 2016-17040.

Burkett, V. S., Cummins, J. M., Dickson, R. M., & Solnick, M. (2005). An open clinical trial utilizing real-time EEG operant conditioning as an adjunctive therapy in the treatment of crack cocaine dependence. *J of Neurotherapy, 9*(2), 27-48.

Burns, D. D. (2008). *Feeling good: The new mood therapy. The clinically proven drug-free treatment for depression.* New York, NY: HarperCollins Publishers.

Bush, N. (2018). *One by one: A memoir of love and loss in the shadows of opioid America.* New York, NY: Apollo Publishers

Butzin, C. A., O'Connell, D. J., Martin, S. S., & Inciardi, J. A. (2006). Effect of drug treatment during work release on new arrests and incarcerations. *Journal of Criminal Justice, 34*(5), 557-565.

Byers, A. P., Forrest, G. G., & Zaccaria, J. (1968). Recalled early parent-child relations, adult needs and occupational choice: A test of Roe's theory. *Journal of Counseling Psychology*, pp. 15, 324-328.

Byers, A. P. (1995). Neurofeedback therapy for a mild head injury. *Journal of Neurotherapy, 1*(1), 22-37.

Cade, C. M., & Coxhead, N. (1989). *The awakened mind: biofeedback and the development of higher states of awareness.* Shaftesbury, Dorset: Element Books.

Carson, R. E. (2012). *The brain fix: What's the matter with your gray matter.* Deerfield Beach, FL: Health Communications, Inc.

Carroll, A. E. (2018). It's time for a new discussion of marijuana's risks. *The New York Times.* Retrieved from https://www.nytimes.com/2018/05/07/upshot/its-time-for-a-new-discussion-of-marijuanas-risks.html

Casey, J., Macri, M., & Davidson, T. (2010, December 19). Increasing rates of post-traumatic stress disorder associated with Iraq and Afghanistan wars. *Project Censored.* Retrieved from https://www.projectcensored.org/increasing-rates-of-post-traumatic-stress-disorder-associated-with-the-iraq-and-afghanistan-wars/

Cass, H. (2015). *The addicted brain: And how to break free.* Marina Del Ray, CA: Better Balance Books.

Cass, H., & Holford, P. (2003). *Natural highs: Supplements, nutrition, and mind-body techniques to help you feel good all the time.* New York, NY: Penguin-Putnam.

Cassani, M. (2013, August 5). Beyond meds Monica Cassani discusses the big picture. Reposted by Rossa Forbes: *Holistic Recovery from Schizophrenia.* https://rossaforbes.com/beyond-meds-monica-cassani-discusses-the-big-picture/

Center for Addiction and Substance Abuse (CASA). (2005, July). *Under the counter: The diversion and abuse of controlled prescription drugs in the US.* Columbia University: New York, NY.

Center for Addiction and Substance Abuse (CASA). (2007, May). *You've got drugs IV: Prescription drug pushers on the internet.* US Senate Judiciary Committee hearing on "Rogue Online Pharmacies". Columbia University: New York, NY.

Center for Behavioral Health Statistics and Quality (2015). *Behavioral health trends in the United States: 2014 national survey on drug use and health.* (HHS Publication No. SMA15-4927, USDUH Series H-50). Retrieved from http://www.samhsa.gov/data/

Chandler, R. K, Fletcher, B. W., & Volkow, N. D. (2009). Treating drug abuse and addiction in the criminal justice system: Improving public health and safety. *Journal of the American Medical Association, 301*(2), 183–190.

Chartier, D. (2017). Alpha-theta training in the treatment of dissociative identity disorder. In A. Martins-Mourao & C. Kerson (Eds.), Alpha-theta neurofeedback in the 21st century A handbook for clinicians and researchers. *Neurofeedback and Neuromodulation Research Foundation*, Murfreesboro, TN. pp. 205-222.

Childs, A., & Price, L. (2007). Cranial electro-therapy stimulation reduces aggression in violent neuropsychiatric patients. *Primary Psychiatry, 14*(3), 50-56.

Choi, S. W., Chi, S. E., Chung, S. Y., Kim, J. W., Ahn, C. Y., & Kim, H. T. (2011). Is Alpha wave neurofeedback effective with randomized clinical trials in depression: A pilot study. *Neuropsychobiology, 63,* 42-51.

Coleman, P. (2006). *Flashback: Posttraumatic stress disorder, suicide, and the lessons of war.* Boston, MA: Beacon Press.

Coleman, P. (2011, April 21). Why are we throwing traumatized vets in jail for calling 911? *AlterNet.* Retrieved from https://www.alternet.org/2011/04/why_are_we_throwing_traumatized_vets_in_jail_for_calling_911/

Compton, W. M. (2018). The need to incorporate smoking cessation into behavioral health treatment. *The American Journal on Addictions, 27*(1), 42–43.

Compton, W. M, & Volkow, N. D. (2006). Major increases in opioid analgesics in the United States: Concerns and suggestions. *Drug Alcohol Dep, 81,* 103-107.

Corry, C. E. (2009). The war against veterans: Why a special court is needed. *Equal Justice Foundation.* Available from http://www.ejfi.org/Courts/Courts-40.htm#50503880_marker-1551751

Corry, C. E. (2010). Iraq veteran suffering from PTSD charged with attempted murder in Colorado Springs. *Equal Justice Foundation.* Available from http://www.ejfi.org/Courts/Courts-42.htm#pgfId-1425559

Corry, C. E. (2010). Veterans court: restorative rather than punitive justice. *Equal Justice Foundation.* Available from http://www.ejfi.org/Courts/Courts-46.htm#pgfId-1425559

Corry, C. E. (2019). Post traumatic stress and injustice. Newsletter. *Equal Justice Foundation*. Available from http://ejfi.org/News/Courts-February_24_2019.htm

Corry, C. E., Stockburger, D. W. (2013, April 22). Analysis of veteran arrests, El Paso County, Colorado. *Equal Justice Foundation*. Available from http://ejfi.org/PDF/EJF_EPCO_vet_arrest_study.pdf

Corry, C. E. (2014). Death of a soldier. *Equal Justice Foundation*. Available from http://www.ejfi.org/Courts/Courts-50.htm#pgfId-1447923

Corry, C. E. (2015). Creating homeless veterans. *Equal Justice Foundation*. Available from http://www.ejfi.org/Courts/Courts-53.htm#pgfId-1447919

Corry, C. E. (2015). Preliminary investigation of veteran deaths in El Paso County, Colorado. *Equal Justice Foundation*. Available from http://www.ejfi.org/Courts/Courts-52.htm#pgfId-1447919

Cottler, L. B., Compton, W. M., Mager, D., Spitznagel, E. L., & Janca, A. (1992). Posttraumatic stress disorder among substance users from the general population. *The American Journal of Psychiatry, 149*(5), 664–670.

Cripe, C. T. (2006). Effective use of LENS unit as an adjunct to cognitive neuro-developmental training. *Journal of Neurotherapy, 10*(2/3), 79-87.

Crist, C. (2019). Healthier diet may help lift depression symptoms. *PLoS*. https://journals.plos.org/plosone/article?id=10.1371/journal.pone.0222768

Cunningham, A. (2019, January 17). Overdose deaths tied to antianxiety drugs like Xanax continue to rise. *Science News*. Retrieved from https://www.sciencenews.org/article/overdose-deaths-tied-antianxiety-drugs-xanax-continue-rise

Cushing, R. E., & Braun, K. L. (2018). Mind-body therapy for military veterans with post-traumatic stress disorder: A systematic review. *Journal of Alternative and Complementary Medicine, 24*(2).

Cushing, R. E., Braun, K. L., et all. (2018). Military-tailored yoga for veterans with post-traumatic stress disorder. *Military Medicine, 183*(5-6), e223-2231.

D'Andrea, W., Ford, J., Stolbach, B., Spinazzola, J., & van der Kolk, B. A. (2012). Understanding interpersonal trauma in children: Why we need a developmentally appropriate trauma diagnosis., American Journal of *Orthopsychiatry, 82*, 187-200.

Davis, R., & Bodenhamer-Davis, E. (2017). Two case studies in outpatient a/t training for trauma. In A. Martins-Mourao & C. Kerson (Eds.), Alpha-theta neurofeedback in the 21st century. *Foundation for Neurofeedback and Neuromodulation Research*, Murfreesboro, TN. pp. 185-204.

deBeus, R. J., Prinzal, H., Ryder-Cook, A., & Allen, L. (2002). QEEG based versus research-based EEG biofeedback treatment with chemically dependent outpatients: Preliminary results. *Journal of Neurotherapy, 6*(1), 54-55.

De Felice, E. A. (1997). Cranial electrotherapy stimulation (CES) in the treatment of anxiety and other stress-related disorders: A review of controlled clinical trials. *Stress Medicine, 13*(1), 31-42.

Dehghani-Arani, F., Rostami, R., & Nadali, H. (2013). Neurofeedback training for opiate addiction: Improvement of mental health and craving. *Applied Psychophysiology & Biofeedback, 38*(2), 133-141.

Del Brutto, O. H., Mera, R. M., Del Brutto, V. J., Maestre, G. E., Gardener, H., Zambrano, M., & Wright, C. B. (2015). Influence of depression, anxiety and stress on cognitive performance in community-dwelling older adults living in rural Ecuador: Results of the Atahualpa Project. *Geriatrics & Gerontology International, 15*(4), 508–514. http://dx.doi.org/10.1111/ggi.12305

Dell, P. F. (2006). The Multidimensional Inventory of Dissociation (MID): A comprehensive measure of pathological dissociation. *Journal of Trauma & Dissociation, 7,* 77-106. doi:10:1300/J229v07n02_06

Demers C. H., Bogdan, R., & Agrawal, A. (2014). The genetics, neurogenetics and pharmacogenetics of addiction. *Curr Behav Neuroscience Rep, 1,* 33-44.

Demos, J. N. (2005). *Getting started with neurofeedback.* New York, NY: W. Norton & Company.

Doidge, N. (2007). *The brain that changes itself: Stories of personal triumph from the frontiers of brain science.* New York, NY: Viking.

Donaldson, C. C. S., Donaldson, S., & Moran, D. (2004). The effect of LENS treatment on cognitive functioning and brainwave patterns. *Biofeedback, 42*(4), 63-68.

DonoVan, B. S., Padin-Rivera, E., Dowd, T., & Blake, D. D. (1996). Childhood factors and war zone stress in chronic PTSD. *Journal of Traumatic Stress, 9,* 361-368.

Drug Policy Alliance. (2020). A brief history of the drug war. Nonprofit: New York, NY. Retrieved from: http://www.drugpolicy.org/issues/brief-history-drug-war

Dubi, M., Powell, P., & Gentry, E. (2017). *Trauma, PTSD, grief & loss: The 10 core competencies for evidence-based treatment.* New York, NY: PESI Publishing.

Duff, J. (2004). The usefulness of quantitative EEG(QEEG) and neurotherapy in the assessment and treatment of post-concussion syndrome. *Clinical EEG & Neuroscience, 35*(4).

Dupont, R. L. (2015, July 1). It's time to re-think prevention; increasing percentages of adolescents understand they should not use any addicting substances. Rockville, MD: *Institute for Behavior and Health, Inc.* Available from www.PreventTeenDrugUse.org

Dupont, R. L., & McClellan, A. T. (2017). Facing addiction in America: The surgeon general's report on alcohol, drug abuse and health: A new agenda to turn back the drug epidemic. Rockville, MD: *Institute for behavior and Health, Inc.* Available from https://www.ibhinc.org/events

Dupont, R. L., McLellan, A. T., White, W. L., Merio, L., & Gold, M. S. (2009). Setting the standard for recovery: Physicians health programs evaluation review. *Journal of Substance Abuse Treatment, 36*(2), 159-171.

Edlund, M., Martin, B. C., Fan, M. Y., Devries, A., Braden, J. B., & Sullivan, M. D. (2010). Risks for opioid abuse and dependence among participants of chronic opioid therapy: Results from the TROUP Study. *Drug Alcohol Dep, 112,* 90-98.

Edwards, E., & McCray, R. (2012, April 26). Hundreds of economists: Marijuana prohibition costs billions, legalization would earn billions. ACLU Blog. https://www.aclu.org/blog/mass-incarceration/hundreds-economists-marijuana-prohibition-costs-billions-legalization-would

Elliott, J. (2016). Sober ever after: A memoir. Amazon.com: Sober Sassy Life.

Emmerson, P., & Hooper, E. (2011). *Overcoming trauma through yoga: Reclaiming your body.* Berkeley, CA: North Atlantic Books.

Erickson, K. (2004). Impact of brain scans: Brain scans could become dominant facet of addiction studies. In K. Stovell & S. Gray (Eds.), *Understanding the addicted brain: From science to science.* Providence, RI: Manisses Communications.

Esty, M. L. (2006). Reflections on FMS treatment, research and neurotherapy: Cautionary tales. *Journal of Neurotherapy, 10*(2/3), 63-68.

Esty, M. L., & Schfflett, C. M. (2014). *Conquering concussion: healing TBI symptoms with neurofeedback and without drugs.* Sewickley, PA: Round Earth Publishing.

Fahrion, S. L., Watson, E. D., Coyne, L., & Allen, T. (1992). Alterations in EEG amplitude, personality factors, and brain electrical mapping after alpha-theta brainwave training: A controlled study of an alcoholic in recovery. *Alcoholism: Clinical and Experimental Research, 16*(3), 547-552.

Figley, C. R. (1978). *Stress disorders among Vietnam veterans.* New York, NY: Brunner/Mazel.

Firth, J., Teasdale, S. B., & Allott, K. (2019). The efficacy and safety of nutrient supplements in the treatment of mental disorders: A meta-review of meta-analysis of randomized controlled trials. *World Psychiatry, 18*(3), 308-324.

Fisher, S. F. (2014). *Neurofeedback in the treatment of developmental trauma: Calming the fear-driven brain.* New York, NY: W. W. Norton.

Fletcher, B. W., & Redonnam-Chandler, J. (2010). *Principles of Drug Abuse Treatment for Criminal Justice Populations - A Research-Based Guide.* The Office of Science Policy and Communications, National Institute on Drug Abuse.

Foote, J., Wilkins, C., Kosanke, N., & Higgs, S. (2014). *Beyond addiction: How science and kindness help people change.* New York, NY: Scribner.

Ford, J. (1999). Disorder of extreme stress following war-zone military trauma: Associated features of posttraumatic stress disorder or comorbid but distinct syndromes. *Journal of Consulting and Clinical Psychology, 67,* 3-12.

Forrest, G. G. (1970). *Transparency as a prognostic variable in psychotherapy* (unpublished doctoral dissertation). U of North Dakota, Grand Forks, ND.

Forrest, G. G. (1979). Negative and positive addictions. Family and Community Health. *The Journal of Health Promotion and Maintenance, 2*(1), 103-113.

Forrest, G. G. (1979, August). Setting alcoholic patients up for therapeutic failure. Family and Community Health: *The Journal of Health Promotion and Maintenance, 2*(1), 69-64.

Forrest, G. G. (1984, August). Psychotherapy of alcoholism and substance abuse: Outcome assessment revisited. Family and Community Health. *The Journal of Health Promotion and Maintenance,* pp. 40-50.

Forrest, G. G. (1983, 1994). *Alcoholism and human sexuality.* Springfield, Charles, C. Thomas; paperback edition, Northvale, NJ: Jason Aronson, Inc.

Forrest, G. G. (1983, 1999). *Alcoholism, narcissism, and psychopathology.* Springfield: Charles C. Thomas; paperback edition, Northvale, NJ: Jason Aronson, Inc.

Forrest, G. G. (1994, 1996). *Chemical dependency and antisocial personality disorder: Psychotherapy and assessment strategies.* Binghamton, NY: Haworth.

Forrest, G. G. (1982, 1992). *Confrontation in psychotherapy with the alcoholic.* Holmes Beach, FL: Learning Publications.

Forrest, G. G. (2002). *Countertransference in chemical dependency counseling.* Binghamton, NY: Haworth Press.

Forrest, G. G. (1975, 1978, 1994). *The diagnosis and treatment of alcoholism.* Springfield: Charles C. Thomas; paperback edition, Northvale, NJ: Jason Aronson, Inc.

Forrest, G. G. (1989, 1994). *Guidelines for responsible drinking.* Springfield, Charles C. Thomas; paperback edition, Northvale, NJ: Jason Aronson, Inc.

Forrest, G. G. (1980, 2001). *How to live with a problem drinker and survive.* New York, NY: Atheneum. Bradenton Beach, FL: Learning Publications.

Forrest, G. G. (2009, 2011). *Self-disclosure in psychotherapy and recovery.* Lanham, MD: Jason Aronson, Inc. Lanham, MD: Rowman & Littlefield Publishers.

Forrest, G. G. (1999-2000). *The Imprisoning of America.* International Academy of Behavioral Medicine Counseling and Psychotherapy (IABMCP) Newsletter Fall/ Winter, 20(1), 3.

Forrest, G. G. (1984, 1997). *Intensive psychotherapy of alcoholism.* Springfield, IL: Charles C. Thomas. Northvale, NJ: Jason Aronson, Inc. [Also, Independent Study Project for Doctor of Philosophy Degree, Columbia Pacific University, San Rafael, CA, January 1984.]

Foster, D. S., & Thatcher, R. W. (2015). Surface and LORETA neurofeedback in the treatment of post-traumatic stress disorder and mild traumatic brain injury. In R. W. Thatcher & D. S. Foster (Eds.), *Z score neurofeedback: Clinical applications* (pp. 59–92). San Diego, CA: Academic Press.

Fragedakis, T. M., Toriello, P. (2014). The Development and experience of combat-related PTSD: a demand for neurofeedback as an effective form of treatment. *Journal of Counseling & Development, 92*(4), 481-488. doi: 10.1002/j.1556-6676.2014.00174.x

Francati, V., Vermetten, E., & Bremmer, J. D. (2007). Functional neuroimaging studies in posttraumatic stress disorder Review of current methods and findings. *Depression & Anxiety, 24*, 202-2018.

France, D. K. L. (2018). *Combat vet don't mean crazy: veteran mental health in post-military life.* Colorado Springs, CO: NCO Historical Society.

Frewen, P. A., & Lundbert, E. (2012). Visual-verbal self/other-referential processing task: Direct vs. Indirect Assessment, variance and experiential correlates. *Personality & Individual Differences, 52*, 509-514. doi:10.1016/J.paid.2011.11.021

Frewen, P., & Lanius, R. (2015). *Healing the traumatized self: Consciousness neuroscience treatment.* Berkeley, CA: Norton Books.

Friedman, M. J. (2010). *Posttraumatic an acute stress disorders* (5th ed.). Sudbury, MA: Jones & Bartlett Learning.

Futures Without Violence. (2020). https://www.futureswithoutviolence.org/

Gambill, G. T. (2008). A mounting social crisis: veterans of Iraq and Afghanistan at the crossroads of justice. Justice Policy Institute. Originally published in *The Daily Journal.* Retrieved from http://www.ejfi.org/Courts/Courts-44.htm

Gant, C, & Lewis, G. (2010). *End your addiction now: The proven nutritional supplement program that can set you free.* Garden City, NY: Square One Publisher.

Gapen, M., van der Kolk, B. A., Hamlin, E., Hirshberg, L., Suvak, M., & Spinazzola, J. (2016). A pilot study of neurofeedback for chronic PTSD. *Applied Psychophysiology and Biofeedback, 41*(3), 251–261. http://dx.doi.org/10.1007/s10484-015-9326-5

Gilham, S., Wild, H., Bayer, Z., Mitchell, M., Sandberg-Lewis, K., & Colbert, A. (2012). Low Energy Neurofeedback System (LENS) for stress, anxiety and cognitive function: An exploratory study. *BMC Complementary and Alternative Med, 12*(Sup. 1), 145.

Gilula, M. F., & Kirsch, D. L. (2005). Cranial electrotherapy stimulation review: A safer alternative to psychopharmaceuticals in the treatment of depression. *Journal of Neurotherapy, 9*(2), 7-26.

Glaser, D. (2000). Child abuse and neglect and the brain: A review. *Journal of Child Psychology and Psychiatry, 19*, 631-657.

Gleick, J. (2008). *Chaos: Making a new science.* New York, NY: Penguin Publishing.

Glenmullen, J. (2000). *Prozac backlash: Overcoming the dangers of Prozac, Zoloft, Paxil, and other antidepressants with safe, effective alternatives.* New York, NY: Simon & Schuster.

Glucek, B. C., & Strobel, C. F. (1975). Biofeedback and meditation in the treatment of psychiatric illness. *Comprehensive Psychiatry, 16*(4), 303-321.

Goldberg, R. J., Greenwood, J., & Taintor, Z. (1976). Alpha conditioning as an adjunct treatment for drug dependence: Part I. *International Journal of Addiction, 11*(6), 1085-1089.

Goldberg, R. J., Greenwood, J., & Taintor, Z. (1977). Alpha conditioning as an adjunct treatment for drug dependence: Part II. *International Journal of Addiction, 12*(1), 195-204.

Goldsmith, L., & Moncrief, J. (2011). The psychoactive effects of antidepressants and their association with suicidality. *Current Drug Safety, 6*(2), 115-121.

Goldstein, R. Z., & Volkow, N. D. (2011). Dysfunction of the prefrontal cortex in addiction: Neuroimaging findings and clinical implications. *Nat Rev Neuroscience, 12*, 652-669.

Gordan, A. J., Wentz, C. M., Gibbon, J. L., Mason, A. D., Freyder, P. J., & O'Toole, T. P. (2002). Relationships between patient characteristics and unsuccessful detoxification. *Journal of Addictive Diseases, 20*(2), 41-53.

Gotsch, K., & Basti, V. (2018, August 2). Capitalizing on mass incarceration: U.S. growth in private prisons. *Incarceration Publication.* Retrieved from: https://www.sentencingproject.org/publications/capitalizing-on-mass-incarceration-u-s-growth-in-private-prisons/

Greene-Shortbridge, T. M., Britt, T. W., & Andrew, C. (2007). The stigma of mental health problems in the military. *Military Medicine, 172*, 157-161.

Greenstein, L. (2017, November 8). PTSD and trauma: Not just for veterans. *National Alliance on Mental Illness.* Retrieved from https://www.nami.org/Blogs/NAMI-Blog/November-2017/PTSD-and-Trauma-Not-Just-for-Veterans

Grin-Yatsenko, V. A., Othmer, S., Pononmarev, V. A., Sergey, S. A., Evdokimov, A., Konoplev, Y. Y., & Konoplev, J. (2018). Infra-low frequency neurofeedback in depression: Thee case studies. *NeuroRegulation, 5*(1), 30-42.

Gross, C. G. (2009). *A hole in the head: Tales in the history of neuroscience.* Cambridge, MA: MIT Press.

Gunkelman, J. (2006). Transcend the DSM using phenotypes. *Biofeedback, 34*(3), 95-98.

Gunkelman, J. (2013). *Explaining Neurofeedback.* Q-Metrx, Inc. Available from www.learningdiscoveries.com

Gunkelman, J. (2017). Alpha/theta training and phenotypes. In A. Martins-Mourao & C. Kerson (Eds.), Alpha-theta neurofeedback in the 21st century A handbook for clinicians and researchers. *Foundation for Neurofeedback and Neuromodulation Research*, Murfreesboro, TN. pp. 173-183.

Gunkelman, J., & Johnstone, J. (2005). Neurofeedback and the brain. *Journal of Adult Development, 12*(2/3), 93-98.

Gunkelman, J., & Cripe, C. (2008). Clinical outcomes in addiction: A neurofeedback case series. *Biofeedback, 36*(4), 152-156.

Hammond, D. C. (2001). Neurofeedback training for anger control. *Journal of Neurotherapy, 5*(4), 98-102.

Hammond, D. C. (2001). Neurofeedback treatment of depression with the Roshi. *Journal of Neurotherapy, 4*(2), 45-56.

Hammond, D. C. (2001). Treatment of chronic fatigue with neurofeedback and self-hypnosis. *Neuro-Rehabilitation, 16*, 295-300.

Hammond, D. C. (2001). QEEG-guided neurofeedback in the treatment of obsessive-compulsive disorder. *Journal of Neurotherapy, 7*(2), 225-32.

Hammond, D. C. (2004). Treatment of the obsessional subtype of obsessive-compulsive disorder with neurofeedback. *Biofeedback, 32*, 9-12.

Hammond, D. C. (2005). Neurofeedback treatment of depression and anxiety. *Journal of Adult Development, 12*, 131-138.

Hammond, D. C. (2005). Neurofeedback to improve physical balance, incontinence and swallowing. *Journal of Neurotherapy, 9*(1), 27-36.

Hammond, D. C. (2005). Neurofeedback with anxiety and affective disorders. *Child & Adolescent Psychiatric Clinics of North America, 14*(1), 105-123.

Hammond, D. C. (2005). Temporal lobes and their importance in neurofeedback. *Journal of Neurotherapy, 9*(1), 67-87.

Hammond, D. C. (2006). *LENS: The Low Energy Neurofeedback System.* Binghamton, NY: The Haworth Press, Inc.

Hammond, D. C. (2006). Introduction: Low energy neurofeedback system: New ideas treatment, and methods. *Journal of Neurotherapy, 10*(2/3), 1.

Hammond, D. C. (2007). Can LENS neurofeedback treat anosmia resulting from a head injury? *Journal of Neurotherapy, 11*(11), 57-62.

Hammond, D. C. (2010). LENS neurofeedback treatment of anger: preliminary reports. *Journal of Neurotherapy, 14*(2), 162-169. http://dx.doi.org/10.1080/10874201003767213

Hammond, D. C. (2010). QEEG evaluation of the LENS treatment of TBI. *Journal of Neurotherapy, 14*(2), 170-177. http://dx.doi.org/10.1080/10874201003767163

Hammond, D. C. (2011). *LENS: The Low Energy Neurofeedback System.* New York: NY: Routledge.

Hammond, D. C. (2011). What is neurofeedback: An update. *Journal of Neurotherapy, 15*, 305-336. http://dx.doi.org/10.1080/10874208.2011.623090

Hammond, D. C. (2012). LENS neurofeedback treatment with fetal alcohol spectrum. *Journal of Neurotherapy, 16*(1), 47-52.

Hammond, D. C., Stockdale, S., Hoffman, D., Ayers, M. E., & Nash, J. (2001). Adverse reactions and potential iatrogenic effects in neurofeedback training. *Journal of Neurotherapy, 4*(4), 57-69.

Hammond, D. C., Walker, J., Hoffman, D., Lubar, J. F., Trudeau, D., Gurnee, R., & Horvat, J. (2004). Standards for the use of quantitative electroencephalography (QEEG) in neurofeedback: A position paper of the International Society for Neuronal Regulation. *Journal of Neurotherapy, 8*(1), 5-27.

Hammond, D. C., & Baehr, E. (2009). Neurofeedback for the Treatment of Depression. Current Status of Theoretical Issues and Clinical Research. *Introduction to Quantitative EEG and Neurofeedback.* doi:10.1016/B978-0-12-374534-7.00012-5.

Hammond, D. C., Bodenhamer-Davis, G., Gluck, G., Stokes, D., Hunt-Harper, S., Trudeau, D., Macdonald, M., Hunt, J., Kirk, L. (2011). Standards of Practice for Neurofeedback and Neurotherapy: A Position Paper of the International Society for Neurofeedback & Research. *Journal of Neurotherapy, 15*(1).

Hammond. D. C., & Gunkelman, J. (2011). *The art of artifacting*. ISNR Research Foundation, San Rafael, CA.

Hammond, D. C., Harper, H., O'Brian, J., & Dorgis, N. (2011, December). Advancement in LENS treatment protocols. *Neuro Connections*, 19-23.

Hanson, G., Venturelli, P. J., & Fleckenstein, A. E. (2017). *Drugs and Society*. Burlington, MA: Jones and Bartlett Learning.

Hari, J. (2015). *Chasing the scream: The first and last days of the war on drugs*. New York, NY: Bloomsbury Publishing.

Hari, J. (2015, September 2). Television Interview. *Chasing the scream: The war on drugs*. Studio10 on Network TEN. Sydney, New South Wales. Available from https://www.youtube.com/watch?v=n37Q68WMtcg

Harper, M. L., Rasolkhani-Kalhorn, T., & Drozd, J. F. (2009). On the neural basis of EMDR therapy: Insights from qEEG studies. *Traumatology*, *15*(2), 81–95. http://dx.doi.org/10.1177/1534765609338498

Harper, S. H. (2009). Low energy neurofeedback system treatment of an acquired brain injury due to sudden cardiac arrest. *Biofeedback*, *37*(3), 100-103.

Harper, S. H., & O'Brien, J. (2011). Two channel low energy neurofeedback system and neurofield with treatment resistant depression: Observations. *NeuroConnections* (Winter), 29-32.

Harrington, T. (2018). Physical trauma diagram. Available from www.echotraining.org

Harvard Health. (2018). *Major depression*. Harvard Medical School. Harvard Health Publishing. Retrieved from https://www.health.harvard.edu/a_to_z/major-depression-a-to-z

Hashemian, P. (2015). The effectiveness of neurofeedback therapy in craving of methamphetamine use. *Open Journal of Psychiatry*, *5*(2), 177.

Haydon, I. (2018). How opioids reshape your brain, and what scientist are learning about addiction. The Philadelphia Inquirer. Retrieved from https//medcalxpress.com/news/2018-opioids-reshape-brain-scientists-addition.html

Heitler, S. (2016). *Prescriptions without pills: For relief from depression, anger, anxiety, and more*. New York, NY: Morgan James Publishing.

Heller, L., & LaPierre, A. (2012). *Healing developmental trauma: How early trauma affects self-regulation, self-image, and the capacity for relationship*. Berkeley, CA: North Atlantic Books.

Helmstetter, S. (2014). *The power of neuroplasticity*. Self Published.

Henderson, C., & Delaney, R. (2017). The price of prisons: Examining state spending trends, 2010–2015, Table 1. Vera Institute of Justice, New York, NY. Available https://www.vera.org/publications/price-of-prisons-2015-state-spending-trends

Henry, G., Woodard, K., Grogan, J. (Producers). (2016--). *60 Days In* [Television Documentary Series]. Jeffersonville, ID: A&E Networks.

Hidasch, B. (2018). *Finishing off the bottle: A memoir of addiction and self-discovery.* Self Published.

Hoemke, S. (2018). *Healing scarred hearts: A family's story of addiction, loss, and finding light.* Dallas, TX: Brown Books Publishing Group.

Hoffman, D. A., Stockdale, S., Hicks, L. L. & Schwaninger, J. E. (1995). Diagnosis and treatment of head injury. *Journal of Neurotherapy, 1*(3), 104-107.

Hoffman, D. A., Stockdale, S., & Van Egen, L. (1996a). EEG Neurofeedback in the treatment of mild traumatic brain injury {Abstract}. *Clinical Electroencephalography, 27*(2), 6.

Hoffman, D. A., Stockdale, S., & Van Egen, L. (1996b). Symptom changes in the treatment of mild traumatic brain injury using EEG neurofeedback {Abstract}. *Clinical Electroencephalography, 27*(2), 164.

Hoffman, G., Koules, O., & Burg, M. (Producers), & Wan, J. (Director). (2004). *Saw* [Motion Picture]. United States: Twisted Pictures.

Hoge, C. W., Castro, C. A., Messer, S. C., McCurk, D., Cotting, D. I., & Koffman, R. L. (2004). Combat duty in Iraq and Afghanistan, mental health problems, and barriers to care. *New England Journal of Medicine, 351*(1), 13-22.

Holleran-Steiker, L. K., Machemehl-Helmly, P., Clements, T., & Earthman, B. (2010). New and promising technologies in the field of addiction recovery: Highlights of emerging benefits. *J of Social Work Practice in the Addictions, 10*(4), 331-338.

Holmes, T., & Holmes, L. (2007). *Parts Work: An illustrated guide to your inner life.* Kalamazoo, MI: Winged Heart Press.

Hooper, J. W., Frewan, P. A., Sack, M., Lanius, R. A., & van der Kolk, B. A. (2007). The responses to script-driven imagery scale (RSDI): Assessment of state post-traumatic symptoms for psychological and treatment research. *Journal of Psychopathology & Behavioral Assessment, 29*(4), 249-268. doi:10.1007/s10862-007-9046-O

Horowitz, S. (2012). Neurofeedback Therapy in clinical applications for cognitive enhancement. *Alternative and Complementary Therapies, 18*(5), 242-247.

Hountras, P. T., & Forrest, G. G. (1970). Personality Characteristics and Self-Disclosure in a Psychiatric Outpatient Population. College of Education Record, *University of North Dakota, 55,* 206-213.

Huang-Storms, L., Bodenhamer-Davis, E., Davis, R., & Dunn, J. (2006). QEEG-Guided neuofeedback for children with histories of abuse and neglect: Neurodevelopmental rationale a pilot study. *J of Neurotherapy, 10*(4), 3-16.

Hughes, S., & Cohen, D. (2009). A systematic review of long-term studies of drug treated and non-drug treated depression. *Journal of Affective Disorders, 118*(1-3), 99-19. https://doi.org/10.1016/j.jad.2009.01.027

Hyman, S. E., & Malenka, R. C. (2001). Addiction and the brain: The neurobiology of compulsion and its persistence. Nature Review Neuroscience, 2(10), 695-703. In (Eds.), A. Martins-Mourao, & C. Kerson, Alpha-theta neurofeedback in the 21st century A handbook for clinicians and researchers. *Neurofeedback and Neuromodulation Research Foundation*, Murfreesboro, TN. pp. 223-244.

Jacobson, L. K., Southwick, S. M., & Kosten, T. R. (2001). Substance use disorders in patients with posttraumatic stress disorder: A review of the literature. *American Journal of Psychiatry, 158*(8), 1184-1190.

Jantz, G. L., & McMurray, A. (2003). *Moving beyond depression: A whole person approach to healing.* Colorado Springs, CO: Waterbrook Press.

Jarvis, M. (2017). Meditation and yoga associated with changes in the brain. *Science, 358*(6362), 461. doi:10.1126/science.358.6362.461

Jarzemboski, W. B. (1985). Electrical stimulation and substance abuse treatment. *Neurobehavioral Toxicology and Teratology, 7*, 119-123.

Johnson, A. R., Kimberly, C., Thibeault, A. J., Lopez, E. D., Peck, K., Sands, P., Sanders, C. M., et all. (2019, January 23). Cues play a critical role in estrous cycle-dependent enhancement of cocaine reinforcement. *Neuropsychopharmacology, 44*, 1189–1197. doi:10.1038/s41386-019-0320-0

Johnson, J. M., & Fox, V. (2018). Beyond thiamine: Treatment for cognitive impairment in Korsakoff's syndrome. *Psychosomatics, 59*(4), 311-317.

Johnson, M., & Davis, E. B. (2017). The therapeutic crossover in a/t training, neurofeedback; temporal and spectral components of access to levels of consciousness. In A. Martins-Mourao & C. Kerson (Eds.), Alpha-theta neurofeedback in the 21st century. *Foundation for Neurofeedback and Neuromodulation Research*, Murfreesboro, TN. pp. 141-172.

Johnstone, J., Gunkelman, J., & Lunt, J. (2005). Clinical database development: characterization of EEG phenotypes. *Clin EEG and Neuroscience, 36*(2), 99-107.

Jones, F. W., & Holmes, D. S. (1976). Alcoholism, alpha production and feedback. *Journal of Consulting and Clinical Psychology, 44*(2), 224-228.

Jones, M., & Hitsman, H. (2018). Neurofeedback treatment for anxiety symptoms. *NeuroRegulation, 5*(3), 85-92.

Journal of Neurotherapy. (2006). Two volume Journal set devoted to the topic of the LENS, 10(2-3), 1-104.

Kang, D. H., Jo, H. J., Jung, W. H., Kim, S. H., Jung, Y. H., Choi, C. H., & Kwon, J. S. (2012). The effect of meditation on brain structure: Cortical thickness mapping and diffusion tensor imaging. *Social Cog and Effective Neuroscience, 8*(1), 27-33.

Kara, O. (2013). The bright future of brain fitness technology. *NeuroConnections* (Winter), 39-46.

Kalechstein, A. D., Newton, T. F., Longshore, D., Anglin, M. D., van Gorp, W. G., & Gawin, F. H. (2000). Psychiatric comorbidity of methamphetamine dependence in a forensic sample. *J of Neuropsychiatry Clinical Neuroscience, 12*(4), 480-484.

Kardiner, A. (1941). *The traumatic neurosis of war.* New York, NY: Paul Hoeber.

Kardiner, A., & Spiegel, H. (1947). *War and neurotic illness.* Oxford, England: Hoeber.

Keith, J. R., Rapgay, L., Theodore, D., Schwartz, J. M., & Ross, J. L. (2015). Assessment of an automated EEG biofeedback system for attention deficits in a substance use disorder residential setting. *Psychology and Addictive Behaviors, 29*(1), 17.

Keller, I. (2001). Neurofeedback Therapy of attention deficits in patients with traumatic brain injury. *Journal of Neurotherapy, 5,* 19-32.

Kelly, M. J. (1997). Native Americans, neurofeedback, and substance abuse theory: Three year outcome of alpha/theta neurofeedback training in the treatment of problem drinking among Dine' (Navajo) people. *J of Neurotherapy, 2*(3), 24-60.

Kerson, C. (2017). The neurophysiology of trauma: Effects on the individual, the body, and the brain. In A. Martins-Mourao & C. Kerson (Eds.), *Alpha-Theta Neurofeedback In the 21st Century.* FNNR, Murfeesboro, TN. pp. 123-139.

Kiluk B. D., & Carroll, K. M. (2013). New developments in behavioral treatments for substance use disorders. *Current Psychiatry Reports, 15,* 420-420.

Kilmer, B., Calkins, J. P., Dupont, R. L., & Humphreys, K. (2017). A large and promising opportunity: reducing substance use in criminal justice populations. In S. C. Miller, D. A. Felin, R. N. Rosenthal, & R. Saitz (Eds.), *The ASAM Principles of Addiction Medicine* (6th ed). Lippincott Williams & Wilkins, Philadelphia, PA.

King, L. A., King, D. W., Fairbank, J. A., Keane, T. M., & Adams, G. A. (1998). Resilience-recovery factors in post-traumatic stress disorder among female and male Vietnam veterans: Hardiness, postwar social support, and additional stressful life events. *Journal of Personality and Social Psychology, 74*(2), 420-34.

Kinslow, F. J. (2008). *The secret of instant healing.* Carlsbad, CA: Hay House.

Kipper, D. (2010). *The addiction solution: Unraveling the mysteries of addiction through cutting-edge brain science.* New York, NY: Rodale.

Kirsch, D. L. (2006). Why electromedicine? *Practical Pain Management, 6*(5), 52-54.

Kluetsch, R. C., Ros, T., Théberge, J., Frewen, P. A., Calhoun, V. D., Schmahl, C., & Lanius, R. A. (2013). Plastic modulation of PTSD resting-state networks and subjective wellbeing by EEG neurofeedback. *Acta Psychiatrica Scandinavica, 130*(2), 123–136. http://dx.doi.org/10.1111/acps.12229

Knishinsky, R. (1998). *The Prozac alternative: Natural relief from depression with St. John's Wort, Kava, Ginkgo, 5-HTP, homeopathy, and other alternative therapies.* Rochester, VT: The Healing Arts Press.

Koob, G. F., & Le Moal, M. (2005). Plasticity of reward neurocircuitry and the 'dark side' of drug addiction. *Nat Neuroscience, 8*, 1442-1444.

Koob, G. F., & Volkow, N. D. (2010). Neurocircuitry of addiction. *Neuropsychopharmacology, 35*, 217-238.

Korsakoff, S. S. (1887). Disturbance of psychic function in alcoholic paralysis and its relation to the disturbance of the psychic sphere in multiple neuritis of nonalcoholic origin (Ob alkogol'nom paraliche). *Vestn Psikhiatrii, 4*(2), 1-102.

Kramer, P. D. (1993). *Listening to Prozac.* New York, NY: Viking Press.

Kranzler, H. R., & Rosenthal, R. N. (2003). Dual diagnosis: Alcoholism and co-morbid psychiatric disorders. *American Journal on Addiction, 12*(S1), S26-S40.

Kravitz, H. M., Esty, M. L., Katz, R. S., Fawcett, J. (2006). Treatment of fibromyalgia syndrome using low-intensity neurofeedback with the flexys neurotherapy system: A randomized controlled trial. *Journal of Neurotherapy, 10*(2/3), 41-58.

Krupitsky E., Nunes, E. V., Ling, W., Gastfriend, D. R., Memisoglu, A., & Silverman, B. L. (2013). Injectable extended-release naltrexone (XR-NTX) for opioid dependence: long-term safety and effectiveness. *Addiction* (Abingdon, England), *108*(9), 1628-1637. doi:10.1111/add.12208

Laibow, R. E., Stubblebine, A. N., Sandground, H., & Bounias, M. (2001). EEG Neurobiofeedback treatment of patients with brain injury: Part 2: Changes in EEG parameters versus rehabilitation. *Journal of Neurotherapy, 5*(4), 45-71.

Langwell, S. (2016). *Beyond recovery: A journey of grace, love, and forgiveness.* DDP.

Lanius, R., & Frewan, P. A. (2015). *Healing the traumatized self: Consciousness neuroscience treatment.* New York, NY: W. W. Norton & Co.

Lanius, R. A., Frewen, P. A., Tursich, M., Jetly, R., & McKinnon, M. C. (2015). Restoring large-scale brain networks in PTSD and related disorders: A proposal for neuroscientifically-informed treatment interventions. *European Journal of Psychotraumatology, 6*(1). http://dx.doi.org/10.3402 /ejpt.v6.27313

Lanius, U. F. (2015). Neurobiology and treatment of traumatic dissociation. Journal Entry. *Personality and Social Psychology, 74*, 420-434.

Larson, S. (2006). *The healing power of neurofeedback: The revolutionary LENS technique for restoring optimal brain function.* Rochester, VT: Healing Arts.

Larson, S., Harrington, K., & Hicks, S. (2006). The LENS (Low Energy Neurofeedback Systems): A clinical outcomes study on one hundred patients at stone mountain center, New York. *Journal of Neurotherapy, 10*(2/3), 69-78.

Larson, S., Larson, R., Hammond, D. C., Sheppard, S., Ochs, L., Johnson, S., Adinaro, C., & Chapman, C. (2006). The LENS neurofeedback with animals, *Journal of Neurotherapy,* 10(2-3), 89-104.

Larson, S. (2009). The special applicability of the low energy neurofeedback system form of neurofeedback to traumatic brain injury: I. The Theory. *Biofeedback, 37*(3), 104-107. https://doi.org/10.5298/1081-5937-37.3.104

Larson, S., Ochs, L., Esty, M. L., & Othmer, S. (2009). Healing the wounds of war and violence: TBI and PTSD with vets and terror survivors. *Journal of Neurotherapy, 13*(4). 269.

Lasser, K., Boyd, J. W., Woolhandler, S., Himmelstein, D. U., McCormick, D., Bor, D. H. (2000). Smoking and mental illness: a population-based prevalence study. *Journal of the American Medical Association, 284*(20), 2606–2610.

Lathan, C., Spira, J. L., Bleiberg, J., Vice, J., & Tsao, J. W. (2013). Defense Automated Neurobehavioral Assessment (DANA): Psychometric properties of a new field-deployable neurocognitive assessment tool. *Military Medicine, 178*(4), 365–371. http://dx.doi.org/10.7205/MILMED-D-12-00438

Lawlis, F., & Martinez, L. (2015). *Psychoneuroplasticity protocols for addictions: A clinical companion for the big book.* Lanham, MD: Rowman & Littlefield.

Laub, D., & Auerhahn, N. C. (1989). Failed empathy: A central theme in the survivor's holocaust experience. *Psychoanalytic Psychology, 6*(4), 377-400. https://doi.org/10.1037/0736-9735.6.4.377

Laufer, R. S. (1988). The serial self: War trauma, identity, and adult development. In J. P. Wilson, Z. Harel, & B. Kahana (Eds.), *The Plenum series on stress and coping.* Human adaptation to extreme stress: From the Holocaust to Vietnam (p. 33–53). Plenum Press.

LeDoux, J. (2015). *The emotional brain: The mysterious underpinnings of emotional life.* New York, NY: Simon and Schuster.

LeDoux, J. (2015). *Anxious: Using the brain to treat fear and anxiety.* New York, NY: Viking Press.

LeDoux, J. (2019). *The deep history of ourselves: The four-billion-year story of how we got conscious brains.* New York, NY: Viking Press.

Lembke, A., Papac, J., & Humphreys, K. (2018, February 22). Our other prescription drug problem. *New England Journal of Medicine, 378*, 693-695. doi:10.1056/NEJMp1715050

Lemonick, M. D. (2019, October). *The science of addiction.* Time Special Edition: The science of addiction, Meredith Corporation, New York, NY.

Leukefeld, C. G., Tims, F., & Farabee, D. (2002). *Treatment of Drug Offenders: Policies and Issues.* Springer, New York, NY.

Levin, F. R., & Kleber, H. D. (1995). Attention-deficit hyperactivity disorder and substance abuse: Relationships and implications for treatment. *Harvard Review of Psychiatry, 2*(5), 246-258.

Levine, P. (1997). *Waking the tiger: Healing trauma.* Berkeley, CA: North Atlantic.

Levine, P. (2010). *In an unspoken voice: How the body releases trauma and restores goodness.* Berkeley, CA: North Atlantic Books.

Levine, P. (2015). *Trauma and memory: Brain and body in a search for the living past.* Berkeley, CA: North Atlantic Books.

Levine, R. A., Walsh, C. A., & Schwartz, R. D. (1996). *Pharmacology: Drug actions and reactions.* New York, NY: Parthenon Publishing Group.

Levy, T. E. (2019). *Magnesium: Reversing disease.* Henderson, NV: MedFox Pub.

Levy, S. J., Williams, J. F., & AAP Committee on Substance Use and Prevention (2016). Substance abuse screening, and intervention and referral to treatment. *Pediatrics, 1338*(1), e20161211.

Liboff, A. R. (2004). Toward an electromagnetic paradigm for biology and medicine. *Journal of Alternative and Complementary Medicine, 10*(1), 41-47.

Lieber, M. (2018). *Equine-assisted therapy may help autism, PTSD and pain. Why isn't it used more?* CNN 2:37 PM ET, Tue July 10, 2018.

Linden, D. J. (2008). *The accidental mind: How brain evolution has given us love, memory, dreams and God.* Cambridge, MA: Belknap Press.

Lopez, G. (2019, January 15). *Americans are now more likely to die from opioid overdose than car crashes.* Vox Media. Retrieved from https://www.vox.com/

Luchins, A. S. (1964). *Group therapy a guide.* (3rd ed.). New York, NY: Random House. OCLC 599119917.

Luciani, A. A. (2001). *Self-coaching: How to heal anxiety and depression.* New York, NY: John Wiley & Sons.

Macready, M. (2012). Opening the doors of perception. *Journal of the National Cancer Institute, 104*, 119-120.

Maher, A. R., et al. (2011). Efficacy and comparative effectiveness of atypical antipsychotic medications for off-label uses in adults: a systematic review and meta-analysis. *Journal of American Medical Association, 306*(12), 1359-1369. doi:10.1001/jama.2011.1360

Malkowics, D., Martinez, D., Morales, J. L., Sterman, M. B., & Kaiser, D. (2009). Intensive neurotherapy facilitates recovery from severe brain injury and seizures. The Institute of Advancement of human potential. *Journal of Neurotherapy.* pp. 254-255. doi:10.1080/108742009033

Maredpour, A., Naderi, F., & Mehrabizadeh, H. M. (2013). Comparing the efficacy of EMDR therapy with prolonged exposure therapy for veterans suffering from chronic PTSD. *Amaghan Danesh, 77*(5), 256-36.

Martin, G., & Johnson, C. L. (2005). The Boys Totem Town Neurofeedback Project: A pilot study of EEG Neurofeedback wit incarcerated juvenile felons. *Journal of Neurotherapy, 93*(3), 71-86.

Martin, P. R., Singleton, C. K., & Hiller-Sturmhofel, S. (2003). The role of thiamine deficiency in alcoholic brain disease. *Alcohol Research & Health, 27*(2), 134-142. Retrieved from https://pubs.niaaa.nih.gov/publications/arh27-2/134-142.htm

Martin, S. S., Butzin, C. A., Saum, C. A., & Inciardi, J. A. (1999). Three-year outcomes of therapeutic community treatment for drug-involved offenders in Delaware: From prison to work release to aftercare. *The Prison Journal, 79*(3), 294–320.

Martins-Mourao, A. (2017). Neurofeedback, brainwaves, and alpha/theta neurofeedback training. In A. Martins-Mourao & C. Kerson (Eds.), Alpha-theta neurofeedback in the 21st century A handbook for clinicians and researchers. *Foundation for Neurofeedback and Neuromodulation Research*, Murfreesboro, TN. pp. 1-52.

Martins-Mourao, A. (2017). The integration of the Peniston protocol: A tool for neurotherapists and psychotherapists. In A. Martins-Mourao & C. Kerson (Eds.), Alpha-theta neurofeedback in the 21st century A handbook for clinicians and researchers. *Foundation for Neurofeedback and Neuromodulation Research*, Murfreesboro, TN. pp. 345-371.

Martins-Mourao, A., & Kerson, C. (2017). Alpha-theta neurofeedback in the 21st century A handbook for clinicians and researchers. *Foundation for Neurofeedback and Neuromodulation Research*, Murfreesboro, TN.

Martins-Mourao, A., & Kerson, C. (2017). Equipment, training, and ethical issues. In A. Martins-Mourao & C. Kerson (Eds.), Alpha-theta neurofeedback in the 21st century A handbook for clinicians and researchers. *Foundation for Neurofeedback and Neuromodulation Research*, Murfreesboro, TN. pp. 373-381.

Maté, G. (2008). *In the realm of hungry ghosts: Close encounters with addiction.* Berkeley, CA: North Atlantic Books.

Maté, G. (2009). *The body says no: Exploring the stress disease connection.* Berkeley, CA: North Atlantic Books.

Mathews, L. J. (1994). *Seven weeks to sobriety: The proven program to fight alcoholism through nutrition.* New York, NY: Ballantine Books.

Maust, D., Lin, L., & Blow, F. (2019, February). Benzodiazepine use and misuse among adults in the United States. *Psychiatric Services, 70*(2), 97-106. doi:10.1176/appi.ps.201800321

May, R. (1977). *The meaning of anxiety.* New York, NY: W.W. Norton.

McCrea, M., Prichep, L., Powell, M. R., Chabot, R., & Barr, W. B. (2010). Acute effects and recover after sport-related concussion: A neurocognitive and quantitative brain electrical activity study. *J of Head Trauma Rehabilitation, 25*, 283-292.

McEwen, B. S. (2002). The neurobiology and neuroendocrinology of stress: Implications for post-traumatic stress disorder from a basic science perspective. *Psychiatric Clinics of North America, 25*, 469-494.

McKee, A. C., Canatu, R. C., Nowinski, C. J., Hedley-Whyte, T., Gravett, B. E., Budson, A. E., & Stern, R. A. (2009). Chronic traumatic encephalopathy in athletes: Progressive tauopathy after repetitive head injury. *Journal of Neuropathology & Experimental Neurology, 68*, 709-735.

McLellan, A. T., Skipper, G. E., Campbell, M. G., & DuPont, R. L. (2008). Five-year outcomes in a cohort study of physicians treated for substance use disorders in the United States. *BMJ, 337*, a203. https://doi.org/10.1136/bmj.a2038

McRenolds, C., Bell, J., & Lincourt, T. M. (2017). Neurofeedback: A non-invasive treatment for symptoms of post-traumatic stress disorder in veterans *NeuroRegulation, 3*(4), 114-124.

Miller, J. A. (2013). *Neurotherapy as an Adjunct therapy for addiction solutions: Neuro recovery model.* (n.p.).

Miller, J. A. (2014). *Nine functions of the prefrontal cortex: LENS training – dysfunctional to functional.* (n.p.).

Miller, J. A. (2019a). *Boots on the ground: Neurotherapy for veterans combatting TBIs, PTSD, anxiety, depression and substance use disorder.* Simla, CO: Self Published.

Miller, J. A. (2019b). *Herding cats: Coordinated alternative therapies for TBIs, PTSD, anxiety, depression and substance use disorder.* Simla, CO: Self Published.

Miller, J. A., & Sisco, T. R. (2020). Wernicke-Korsakoff Syndrome (WKS): A case study. *The International Journal of Healing and Caring, 20*(1), 1-16. www.ijhc.org/wernicke-korsakoff-syndrome-wks-context-process-and-a-case-study

Minozzi S., Amato, L., Vecchi, S., Davoli, M., Kirchmayer, U., & Verster, A. (2011). Oral naltrexone maintenance treatment for opioid dependence. *Cochrane Database Syst Rev, 4.* doi:10.1002/14651858.CD001333.pub4

Moncrieff, J. (2001). Are antidepressants overrated? A review of methodological problems in antidepressant trials. *The Journal of Nervous & Mental Disease, 189*(5), 288-205.

Moncrieff, J. (2007). Are antidepressants as effective as claimed? No, they are not effective at all. *Can J Psychiatry, 52*, 96-97.

Moncrieff, J. (2007). Understanding psychotropic drug action: The contribution of the brain disabling theory. *Ethical Human Psychology and Psychiatry, 9*(3), 107.

Moncrieff, J. (2013). Against the stream: Antidepressants are not antidepressants: An alternative approach to drug action and implications for the use of antidepressants. *B. J. Psych Bulletin, 42*(1), 42-44.

Moncrieff, J., & Cohen, D. (2006) Do antidepressants cure or create abnormal brain states? *PLoS Med, 3*(7), e240. https://doi.org/10.1371/journal.pmed.0030240

Moncrieff, J., Cohen, D., & Porter, S. (2013). Medication: The elephant in the room. *Journal of Psychoactive Drugs, 45*(5), 409-415.

Moore, A., & Malinowski, P. (2009). Meditation, mindfulness and cognitive flexibility. *Consciousness and Cognition, 18*(1), 176-186. Available from https://www.ncbi.nlm.nih.gov/pubmed/19181542

Moore, N. C. (2000). A review of EEG biofeedback treatment of anxiety disorders. *Clinical Electroencephalography, 31*(1), 1-6.

Moore, T. J., & Mattison, D. R. (2017, February). Adult utilization of psychiatric drugs and differences by age, sex, and race. *JAMA Internal Medicine, 177*(2), 274-275.

Mooney, A. J., Dold, C., & Eisenberg, H. (2014). *The recovery book: Answers to all your questions about addiction and alcoholism and finding health and happiness in sobriety.* New York, NY: Workman Publishing Company.

Morris, C. (2019, January 21). *Study recommends acupuncture as alternative to opioids.* WSMV. Meredith Corporation. Retrieved from https://www.wsmv.com/news/study-recommends-acupuncture-as-alternative-to-opioids/article_5f203610-1db9-11e9-a7b5-5b39b9979c24.html

Moynihan, R., & Cassels, A. (2005). *Selling sickness: How the world's biggest pharmaceutical companies are turning us all into patients.* New York, NY: Nation.

Mourao, A., & Kerson, C. (Eds). Alpha-theta neurofeedback in the 21st century A handbook for clinicians and researchers. *Foundation for Neurofeedback and Neuromodulation Research,* Murfreesboro, TN. pp. 317-344.

Munn, J. (2019). *Staying sober without God: The practical 12 steps to long-term recovery from alcoholism and addictions.* Self Published.

Nash, J. (2017). Alpha/theta training as a "state access" process. In A. Martins-Mourao & C. Kerson (Eds.), Alpha-theta neurofeedback in the 21st century

A handbook for clinicians and researchers. *Foundation for Neurofeedback and Neuromodulation Research*, Murfreesboro, TN. Pp. 107-121.

National Institute of Mental Health (2016). *Eating Disorders*. Retrieved from https://www.nimh.nih.gov/health/topics/bipolar-disorder/index.shtml

National Institute of Mental Health (2016). *Social anxiety disorder: More than just shyness*. NIH Publication No. 19-MH-8083. U.S. Department of Health and Human Services. Retrieved from: https://www.nimh.nih.gov/health/publications/social-anxiety-disorder-more-than-just-shyness/index.shtml

National Institute on Alcohol Abuse and Alcoholism. (2000, June). The Neurotoxicity of Alcohol. Chapter 2: Alcohol and the Brain. *Neuroscience and Neurobehavior report to U.S. Congress on Alcohol and Health*, 134-146. Retrieved from https://pubs.niaaa.nih.gov/publications/10report/chap02e.pdf

National Institute on Alcohol Abuse and Alcoholism. (2019). Alcohol's damaging effects on the brain. *Alcohol Alert*, 63, 1-6. Retrieved from https://pubs.niaaa.nih.gov/publications/aa63?aa63.htm

NCSL. (2018, July). Barriers to work: People with criminal records. National Conference of State Legislatures. Available from https://www.ncsl.org/research/labor-and-employment/barriers-to-work-individuals-with-criminal-records.aspx

Nelson, D. V., & Esty, M. L. (2009). Neurotherapy for pain in veterans with trauma spectrum disorders. *Journal of Pain*, 10(4), Supplement S18. http://www.jpain.org/article/S1526-5900%2890%29000090-X/abstract

Nelson, D. V., & Esty, M. L. (2012). Neurotherapy of traumatic brain injury/posttraumatic stress symptoms of OEF/OIF veterans. *Journal of Neuropsychiatry and Clinical Neurosciences*, 24(2), 237-240.

Nelson, D. V., & Esty, M. L. (2015). Neurotherapy of traumatic brain injury/post-traumatic stress symptom in Viet Nam veterans. *Military Medicine*, 180, e1111-1114.

Nelson, D.V., & Esty, M. L. (2015). Neurotherapy for chronic headache following traumatic brain injury. *Military Medical Research*, 2(1), 1-5. http://link.springer.com/article/10.1186/s40779-01-0049-y

Nelson, L. A. (2003). Neurotherapy and the challenge of empirical support: A call for a neurotherapy practice research network, *Journal of Neurotherapy*, 2, 33-67.

NeuroScience, Inc. (2010). Pro-grade brand delivering premium products containing amino acids, botanicals, vitamins, and minerals exclusively to thousands of licensed healthcare providers. Available from at http://www.neurorelief.com

Newberg, A., & d'Aquili, E. G. (2008). *Why God won't go away: Brain science and the biology of belief*. New York, NY: Random House, LLC.

NIDA. (2006, July 24). *NIDA announces recommendations to treat drug abusers, save money and reduce crime.* News Release. National Institutes of Health, Chicago, IL. Retrieved from https://www.nih.gov/news-events/news-releases/nida-announces-recommendations-treat-drug-abusers-save-money-reduce-crime

NIDA. (2010, August). *Drugs, brains, and behavior: the science of addition.* Pub.10-5605. Available from http:/www.drugabuse.gov/publications/science-addiction

NIDA. (2012, January). *Why do professionals at risk for losing their licenses continue abusing drugs/alcohol.* NIDA Drug Pubs. Available from http://www.nida.nih.gov/PODAT_CJ/faqs/faqs1.html#6

NIDA. (2014, April 18). *Principles of drug abuse treatment for criminal justice populations - A research-based guide.* Available from https://www.drugabuse.gov/publications/principles-drug-abuse-treatment-criminal-justice-populations-research-based-guide

NIDA. (2015, June 12). *Addiction is a disease of free will.* National Institute on Drug Abuse website. Retrieved November 28, 2019 from https://www.drugabuse.gov/about-nida/noras-blog/2015/06/addiction-disease-free-will

NIDA. (2018, March 23). *What does it mean when we call addiction a brain disorder?* NIH. Available from https://www.drugabuse.gov/about-nida/noras-blog/2018/03/what-does-it-mean-when-we-call-addiction-brain-disorder

NIDA. (2019). Biography of Dr. Nora Volkow. NIH. Retrieved from: https://www.drugabuse.gov/about-nida/directors-page/biography-dr-nora-volkow

Nijenus, E. R., Spinhoven, P., van Dyck, R., Hart, R., & Vanderlinden, J. (1996). The development and psychometric characteristics of the Somatoform Dissociation Questionnaire (SDQ-20). *Journal of Nervous and Mental Disease, 184,* 688-694.

Nikolakaros, G., et al. (2019). A patient with Korsakoff's syndrome of psychiatric and alcoholic etiology presenting as DSM-5 mild neurocognitive disorder. *Neuropsychiatric Disease and Treatment, 15,* 1311-1320. doi:10.2147/NDT.S203513

Noldy, N. E., Santos, C. V., Politzer, N., Blair, R. D., & Carlin, P. L. (2004). Changes in cocaine withdrawal: Evidence for log-term CNS effects. *Neurophysiology, 30*(4), 189-196.

Nunes E. V., Krupitsky, E., Ling, W., et al. (2015). Treating opioid dependence with injectable extended-release naltrexone (XR-NTX): Who will respond? *Journal of Addiction Medicine, 9*(3):238-243. doi:10.1097/ADM.0000000000000125

O'Brian, W. (2015). *Love our vets: Restoring hope for families of veterans with PTSD.* Sisters, OR: Deep River Books, LLC.

O'Brien, C. P., Charney, D. S., Lewis, L., Cornish, J. W., Post, M. R., Woody, G. E., & Bowden, C. L. (2004). Priority actions to improve the care of persons with co-occurring substance abuse and other mental disorders: A call to action. *Biological Psychiatry, 56*(10), 703-713.

Ochs, L. (1994). New light on lights, sounds, and the brain. Megabrain Report. *The Journal of Mind Technology, 2940*, 48-52.

Ochs, L. (1994a). *EEG-Driven stimulation and heterogeneous head injured patients extended findings.* A peer-reviewed abstract from the 1994 Berrol Head Injury Conference, Las Vegas NV. {web page, cited March 15, 2000} Available from http://www.flexyx.com/contents/pubs/Extended.htm

Ochs, L. (1994b). *EEG-Driven stimulation and mild head injured patients: Preliminary findings.* A peer-reviewed abstract from the 1994 Berrol Head Injury Conference, Salt Lake City, UT. {web page, cited March 15, 2000} Available from http//www.flexyx.com/contents/pubs/Preliminary.htm

Ochs, L. (1996). *Thoughts about EEG-Driven stimulation after three years of its uses: Ramifications for concepts of pathology, recovery, and brain function.* Unpublished manuscript.

Ochs, L. (1997). *EDS: Background and operation. EEG-driven pico-photic stimulation.* Walnut Creek, CA: Flexys, LLC.

Ochs, L. (2006a). The low energy neurofeedback system (LENS): Theory, background, and introduction. *Journal of Neurotherapy, 10*(2-3), 5-39.

Ochs, L. (2006b). The low energy neurofeedback system (LENS): Theory, background, and introduction. In D. C. Hammond (Ed.), *LENS: The low energy neurofeedback system.* Binghamton, NY: Hawthorn Medical Press.

Ochs, L. (2006). Comment on the treatment of fibromyalgia syndrome using low-intensity neurofeedback with the flexyx neurotherapy system: A randomized controlled trial, or how to go crazy over nearly nothing. *Journal of Neurotherapy, 10*(2/3) 59-61.

Ochs, L. (2011). Working with traumatic brain injury using the low energy neurofeedback system (the LENS). *Neuroconnections* (Winter), pp. 23-26.

Ochs, L., & Matheis, R. J. (2001). Flexyx neurotherapy system I the treatment of traumatic brain injury: An initial evaluation. *Journal of Head Trauma Rehabilitation, 16*(3), 260-274.

O'Connor, R. (1997). *Undoing depression: what therapy doesn't teach. you and medication can't give you.* New York, NY: Berkeley Books.

Office of National Drug Control Policy. (2013). *Strengthening Military Families and Veterans.* President Barack Obama. Available from https://obamawhitehouse.archives.gov/ondcp/military-veterans

Ogden, P., & Fisher, J. (2015). *Sensorimotor psychotherapy: Interventions for trauma and attachment.* Berkeley, CA: Norton Books.

Ogden, P. (2013). Technique and beyond: Therapeutic enactments, mindfulness, and the role of the body. In D. J. Seigel & M. S. Solomon (Eds.), *Healing moments in psychotherapy*. New York, NY: Norton.

Ogden, P. (2009). Emotion, mindfulness, and movement: Expanding the regulatory boundaries of the window of tolerance. In D. Fosha, D. Siegel, & M. Solomon (Eds.), *The healing power of emotion: Perspectives from affective neuroscience and clinical practice* (pp. 204-231). New York, NY: Norton.

Ogden, P., Minton, K., & Pain, C. (2006). *Trauma and the body: A sensorimotor approach to psychotherapy*. Berkeley, CA: Norton Books.

Ogden, P., Minton, K. (2000). Sensorimotor psychotherapy: One method for processing traumatic memory. *Traumatology, 63*(30), 1-20.

O'Hare, T., Shen, C., & Sherrer, M. (2010). High-risk behaviors and drinking-to-cope as mediators of lifetime abuse and PTSD symptoms in clients with severe mental illness. *Journal of Traumatic Stress, 23*, 255-263.

Ortigas, J. (June, 2013). Carbohydrates trigger the addiction regions of the brain. *Guardian Liberty Voice*. Available from https://guardianlv.com/2013/06/carbohydrates-trigger-the-addiction-regions-of-the-brain/

Oscar-Berman, M., & Marinkovic, K. (2003). Alcoholism and the brain: An overview. *Alcohol Health & Research World, 27*, 125-133.

Oscar-Berman, M., Sagrin, B., Evert, D. L., & Epstein, C. (1997). *Alcohol Health & Research World, 21*(1), 65-121.

Othmer, S., & Steinberg, M. (2010). EEG neurofeedback therapy. In D. Brizer & R. Castaneda (Eds.), *Clinical Addiction Psychiatry,* (pp. 169-187). Cambridge UP.

Packard, R. C., Ham, L. P. (1997). EEG biofeedback for post-traumatic Headache and Cognitive Dysfunction: A Pilot Study. *Headache Q, 8*, 348-352.

Pape, T. L., Rosenow, J., & Lewis, G. (2006). Transcranial magnetic stimulation: a possible treatment for TBI. *J of Head Trauma Rehabilitation, 21*, 437–451.

Passini, F. T., Watson, C. G., Dehnel, L., Herder, J., & Watkins, B. (1977) With alcohol and other drug abuse: Results from the epidemiologic catchment area (ECA) study. *JAMA, 264*(19), 2511-2518.

Paul, L. K., Brown, W. S., Adolphs, R., Tyszka, J. M., Richards, L. J., Mukherjee, P., & Sherr, S. H. (2007). Agenesis of the corpus callosum: genetic, developmental and functional aspects of connectivity. *Nature Reviews Neuroscience, 8*(4), 287-299.

Paulsen, S. (2009). *Looking through the eyes of trauma and dissociation: An illustrated guide for EMDR therapists and clients*. Self Published.

Pavlenko, V. B., Chernyi, S. V., & Goubkina, D. G. (2009). EEG correlates of anxiety and emotional stability in adult healthy subjects. *Neurophysiology, 41*(5), 337–345. http://dx.doi.org/10.1007/s11062-010-9111-2

Peper, E., & Harvey, R. (2018). Digital addiction: Increased loneliness, anxiety, and depression. *NeuroRegulation, 5*(1), 3-8.

Peniston, E. G., & Kulkosky, P. J. (1989). Alpha-theta brainwave training and beta-endorphin levels in alcoholics. *Alcohol: Clin & Exp Research, 13,* 271-279.

Peniston, E. G., & Kulkosky, P. J. (1991). Alcoholic personality and alpha-theta brainwave training. *Medical Psychotherapy, 2,* 37-55.

Peniston, E. G., & Kulkosky, P. J. (1991). Alpha-Theta brainwave neurofeedback therapy for Vietnam veterans with combat-related post-traumatic stress disorder. *Medical Psychotherapy, 4,* 47-60.

Peniston, E. G., Marrinan, D. A., Deming, W. A., & Kulkosky, P. J. (1993). EEG alpha-theta brainwave synchronization in Vietnam theater veterans with combat-related post-traumatic stress disorder and alcohol abuse. *Advances in Medical Psychotherapy, 6,* 37–50.

Pennock, P. E. (2007). *Advertising sin and sickness: The politics of alcohol and tobacco marketing 1950-1990.* DeKalb, IL: Northern Illinois University Press.

Pert, C. (1997). *Molecules of emotion: The science behind mind-body medicine.* New York, NY: Scribner.

Pert, C. (2006). *Everything you need to know to feel good.* Carlsbad, CA: Hay House.

Pert, C. (2013). In the Name of Newtown's children, let's stop the shootings. A psychopharmacologist speaks. Magic Bullets. Retrieved from http://candacepert.com/blog/ | Article No Longer Available.

Prah, P., Petersen, I., Nazareth, I., Walters, K., & Osborn, D. (2011). National changes in oral antipsychotic treatment for people with schizophrenia in primary care between 1998 and 2007 in the United Kingdom. *Pharmacoepidemology and Drug Safety, 21*(2), 161-169. https://doi.org/10.1002/pds.2213

Precourt, A., Dunewicz, M., Grégoire, G., & Williamson, D. R. (2005). Multiple complications and withdrawal syndrome associated with Quetiapine/ Venlafaxine intoxication. *Annals of Pharmacotherapy, 39*(1), 153-156. https://doi.org/10.1345/aph.1E073

Prochaska J. J., Da, S., & Young-Wolff, K. C. (2017). Smoking, mental illness, and public health. *Annu Rev Public Health, 38,* 165–185. doi:10.1146/annurev-publhealth-031816-044618

Procyk, A. (2018). *Nutritional treatments to improve mental health disorders: Non-pharmaceutical interventions for depression, anxiety, bipolar and ADHD.* Eau Claire, WI: PESI Publishing.

Putnam, J. A. (2001). EEG biofeedback on a female stroke victim with depression: A case study. *Journal of Neurotherapy, 5*(3), 27-38.

Quirk, D. A. (1995). Composite biofeedback conditioning and dangerous offenders III. *Journal of Neurotherapy, 1*(2), 44-54.

Raab, D. M., & Brown, J. (2012). *Writers on the edge: 22 writers speak about addiction and dependency.* Ann Arbor, MI: Loving Healing Press.

Raloff, J. (2010, June 22). Abuse of pharmaceuticals is rising sharply. *Science News.* Available from https://www.sciencenews.org/blog/science-the-public/abuse-pharmaceuticals-rising-sharply

Ramachandran, V. S., & Blakeslee, S. (1999). *Phantoms in the brain: Probing the mysteries of the human mind.* New York, NY: Harper Perennial.

Ramel, W., Goldin, P. R., Carmona, P. E., & McQuaid, J. R. (2004). The effects of mindfulness meditation on cognitive processes and affect in patients with past depression. *Cognitive Therapy and Research, 28*(4), 433-455.

Rappoport, J. (2012). Meds killing soldiers by heart attacks. Blog. Available https://blog.nomorefakenews.com/2012/03/30/meds-killing-soldiers-by-heart-attack/

Rasmussen, J. G. C. (1999). Use and misuse: Antidepressants in psychiatric practice. *International Journal of Psychiatry in Clinical Practice, 3*(2), 121-128.

Ray, O., & Ksir, C. (1996). *Drugs, society and human behavior.* St. Louis, MO: Mosby.

Regier, D. A., Farmer, M. E., Rae, D. S., et al. (1990). Comorbidity of Mental Disorders With Alcohol and Other Drug Abuse: Results From the Epidemiologic Catchment Area (ECA) Study. *Journal of the American Medical Association, 264*(19), 2511–2518. doi:10.1001/jama.1990.03450190043026

Retallick–Brown, H. (2020, February). *UC study supports use of nutrients in treatment of PMS.* University of Canterbury. https://www.canterbury.ac.nz/

Richter K. P., & Arnsten, J. H. (2006). A rationale and model for addressing tobacco dependence in substance abuse treatment. *Substance Abuse Treatment, Prevention and Policy, 1*(1), 23.

Riggio, G. (2019, April 21). How the body responds to synthetic THC product 'Spice'. SciWorthy, Blue Marble Space. Retrieved from: https://sciworthy.com/how-the-body-responds-to-spice/

Robbins, J. (2013). *A symphony in the brain: the evolution of the new brain wave neurofeedback.* New York, NY: Grove Press.

Robertson, M., & Tremble, M. R. (1982). Major tranquilizers used as antidepressants: A review. *Journal of Affective Disorders, 4*(3), 173-193. https://doi.org/10.1016/0165-0327(82)90002-7

Robinson, T. E., & Berridge, K. C. (2001). Incentive-sensitization and addiction. *Addiction, 96*(1), 103-114.

Roemer, T. E., Cornwell, A., Dewart, D., Jackson, P., & Ercegovac, D. V. (1995). Quantitative electroencephalographic analysis in cocaine-preferring polysubstance abusers during abstinence. *Psychiatric Research, 58*(31), 247-257.

Roberts, D. (April, 2013). Every mass shooting shares one thing in common, & it's NOT weapons. *Ammo Land.* Opinion. http://www.ammoland.com/

Rosborough, B. (2018). *Emotional recovery from trauma, tragedy and PTSD.* Self Published.

Ross, C. A. (1989). *Multiple personality disorder diagnosis, clinical features and treatment.* New York, NY: John Wiley.

Ross, C. A. (2004). *Schizophrenia: Innovations in diagnosis and treatment.* New York, NY: Hawthorn Press.

Ross, C. A. (2004). *Spirit power drawings: The foundation of a new science.* Richardson, TX: Manitou Communications, Inc.

Ross, C. A. (2005). A proposed trial of dialectical behavior therapy and trauma model therapy. *Psychological Reports, 96*(3), 901-911.

Ross, C. A. (2007). *The CIA doctors: Human rights violations by American Psychiatrists.* Richardson, TX: Manitou Communications, Inc.

Ross, C. A. (2007a). *The trauma model: A solution to the problem of comorbidity in psychiatry.* Richardson, TX: Manitou Communications, Inc.

Ross, C. A. (2007b). *Moon shadows: Stories of traumas and recovery.* Richardson, TX: Manitou Communications, Inc.

Ross, C. A. (2008). *The great psychiatry scam: One shrink's personal journey.* Richardson, TX: Manitou Communications, Inc.

Ross, C. A, (2009). *Military mind control: A story of trauma and recovery.* Richardson, TX: Manitou Communications, Inc.

Ross, C. A. (2013). *Structural dissociation: A proposed modification of the theory.* Richardson, TX: Manitou Communications, Inc.

Ross, C. A. (2016). Trauma model therapy: A treatment approach for traumatized adolescents. *Counselor, 17,* 60-66.

Ross. C. A., & Elliason, J. W. (2001). Acute stabilization in a trauma program. *Journal of Trauma and Dissociation, 2*(2), 83-87.

Ross, C. A., & Haley, C. (2004). Acute stabilization and three-month follow-up in a trauma program. *Journal of Trauma and Dissociation, 5*(1), 103-112.

Ross, C. A., & Burns, S. (2007). Acute stabilization in a trauma program: pilot study. *Journal of Psychological Trauma, 6*(1), 21-8.

Ross, C. A., & Halpern, N. (2009). *Trauma model therapy: A treatment approach for therapy, dissociation and complex comorbidity.* Richardson, TX: Manitou.

Ross, C. A., & Fung, H. W. (2019). *Be a teammate with yourself: Understanding trauma and dissociation.* Richardson, TX: Manitou Communications, Inc.

Ross, J. (2002). *The mood cure: The 4-step program to take charge of your emotions today.* New York, NY: Penguin Books.

Ross, J. (2017). *The craving cure: Identify your craving type to achieve your natural cranial function.* New York, NY: Boric.

Ross, R. J., Cole, M., Thompson, J. S., & Kim, K. H. (1983). Emotional computer tomography EEG and neurological evaluation. *Journal of the American Medical Association, 249,* 211-213.

Ross, S. M. (2017). Microbiota-Gut-Brain axis, Part 1: An integrated system of immunological, neural, and hormonal signals. *Hol Nurs Prac, 31*(2), 133–136.

Ross, S. M. (2019). Natural health strategies for pain care, Part I: A phytomedicine compendium. *Holistic Nursing Practice, 33*(1), 60–65.

Russo, G. M., & Nivian, D. A. (2014). A research analysis of neurofeedback protocols for PTSD and alcoholism. *NeuroRegulation, 1*(2), 183-186.

Rostami, R., & Dehngani-Arani, F. (2015). Neurofeedback training as a method in treatment of crystal methamphetamine dependent patients: A preliminary study. *Applied Psychophysiology & Biofeedback, 40*(3), 151-161.

Rudd, R. A., Seth, P., David, F., & Scholl, L. (2016). Increases in drug and opioid-involved overdose deaths – United States. *M & M Weekly Report, 65*(50-51), 1445-1452. https://www.cdc/mmwr/volumes/65/wr/mm6505l.htm

Sahley, B. J., & Birkner, K. M. (2004). *Break your prescribed addiction: A guide to coming off tranquilizers, antidepressants, SSRIs, & more using amino acids and nutrients.* San Antonio, TX: Pain & Stress Publications.

Salam, A. (2017, October 26). The opioid epidemic: A crisis years in the making. *The New York Times.* Available from https://www.nytimes.com/2017/10/26/us/opioid-crisis-public-health-emergency.html

SAMHSA. (2005). *Substance abuse treatment for persons with co-occurring disorders. Treatment Improvement Protocol* (TIP). Series. No. 42, Ch. 9: Substance-Induced Disorders. National Center for Biotechnology Information, U.S. National Lib of Medicine. Rockville, MD. https://www.ncbi.nlm.nih.gov/books/NBK64178/

SAMHSA. (2014). *Opioid overdose toolkit.* Rockville, MD. Substance Abuse Mental Health Services Administration, US. Dept. of Health and Human Services.

SAMHSA (2017). *Tobacco and behavioral health: The issue and resources.* Rockville, Maryland. Available from https://www.samhsa.gov/sites/default/files/topics/alcohol_tobacco_drugs/tobacco-behavioral-health-issue-resources.pdf

Saxby, E., & Peniston, E. G. (1995). Alpha-theta brainwave neurofeedback training: An effective treatment for male and female alcoholics with depressive symptoms. *Journal of Clinical Psychology, 51*(5), 685-693.

Seal, K., Shi, Y., Cohen, G., Maguen, S., Krens, E. E., & Neylan, T. C. (2012). Association of mental health disorders with prescription opioids and high-risk opioid use in US veterans of Iraq and Afghanistan. *JAMA, 307*(9), 940-947.

Sederer, L. I. (2019). What does "rat park" teach us about addiction? *Psychiatric Times.* Available from https://www.psychiatrictimes.com/substance-use-disorder/what-does-rat-park-teach-us-about-addiction

Schoenberger, N. E., Shiflett, S. C., Esty, M. L., Ochs, L., & Mathesis, R. J. (2001). Flex neurotherapy system in the treatment of traumatic brain injury: An Initial Evaluation. *The Journal of Head Trauma Rehabilitation, 16*(3), 260-274.

Schwartz, A., & Malmberger, B. (2018). *EMDR therapy and somatic psychology: interventions to enhance embodiment in trauma treatment.* New York, NY: W. W. Norton & Company.

Scott, W. C. (2017). Alpha/theta training applied to substance abuse and post-traumatic stress disorder. In A. Martins-Mourao & C. Kerson (Eds.), Alpha-theta neurofeedback in the 21st century A handbook for clinicians and researchers. *Foundation for Neurofeedback and Neuromodulation Research,* Murfreesboro, TN. pp. 281-315.

Scott, W. C., & Kaiser, D. (1998). Augmenting chemical dependency treatment with neurofeedback training. *Journal of Neurotherapy, 3*(1), 455-469.

Scott, W. C., & Kaiser, D. (1998). Augmenting chemical dependency treatment with neurofeedback training. *Journal of Neurotherapy, 3*(1), 66.

Scott, W. C., Kaiser, D., Othmer, S., & Siderhoff, S. L. (2005). Effects of an EEG biofeedback protocol on a mixed substance abusing population. *The American Journal of Drug and Alcohol Abuse, 31*(3), 455-469.

Shapiro, F. (2001). *Eye movement desensitization and reprocessing: Basic principles, protocols, and procedures.* New York, NY: Guilford Press.

Shimer, P. (2004). *Healing secrets of the Native Americans: Herbs, remedies, and practices that restore the body, mind, and spirit.* New York, NY: Tess Press.

Siegel, D. J. (2003). An interpersonal neurobiology of psychotherapy: The developing mind and the resolution of trauma. In M. Solomon & D. Siegel (Ed.), *Healing trauma: Attachment, mind, body, and brain.* (pp. 1-56). New York, NY: Norton.

Siegel, D. J. (2007). *The mindful brain: Reflection and attunement in the culmination of well-being.* New York, NY: W. W. Norton & Co.

Seigel, D. J. (2010). *Mindsight: The new science of personal transformation.* New York, NY: Random House.

Siegel, D. J. (2010, 2012). *The mindful therapist: A clinician's guide to mindsight and neural integration*. New York, NY: W. W. Norton & Co.

Singh, A. (2018). *Medicalizing addiction*. Freedom Magazine. Retrieved https://www.freedommag.org/magazine/201704-addiction/medicalizing-addiction.html

Smith, D. A., & Sams, M. W. (2005). Neurofeedback with juvenile offenders: A pilot study in the use of QEEG-based and analog-based remedial neurofeedback training. *Journal of Neurotherapy, 9*(3), 87-99.

Smith, W. D. (2008). *The effect of neurofeedback training on PTSD symptoms of depression and attention problems among military veterans*. Capella University. Retrieved from http://gradworks.umi.com/33/15/3315214.html

Snyder, C. R., Harris, C., Anderson, J. R., et al. (1991). The will and the ways: Development and validation of an individual-differences measure of hope. *Journal of Personality and Social Psychology, 60*(4), 570–585.

Snyder, P. (2010). *Drugs and the brain*. New York, NY: Freeman & Company.

Sokhadze, T. (2017). Lessons learned from Peniston's brainwave training protocol. In A. Martins-Mourao & C. Kerson (Eds.), Alpha-theta neurofeedback in the 21st century: A handbook for clinicians and researchers. *Neurofeedback and Neuromodulation Research Foundation*, Murfreesboro, TN. pp. 245-279.

Sokhadze, T., Cannon, R., & Trudeau, D. (2008). EEG biofeedback as a treatment for substance use disorders: Review, rating of efficacy and recommendations for further research. *Applied Psychophysiology & Biofeedback, 33*, 1-28.

Sokhadze, E. M., Tradeau, D. L., & Cannon, R. L. (2013). Treating addiction disorders in clinical neurotherapy-applications of techniques for treatment. In D. Cantor & J. Evans (Eds.). *Chemical Neurotherapy*. San Diego, CA: Elsevier.

Sokhadze, E. M., Cowan, J., Tasman, A., Sokhadze, G., Horrell, T., & Stewart, C. (2010). Effects of gamma neurofeedback training on perceived positive emotional state and cognitive functions. *Journal of Neurotherapy, 14*, 343-345.

Sokhadze, E. M., Cannon, R. L., & Trudeau, D. L. (2008). EEG biofeedback as a treatment for substance use disorders: Review, rating of efficacy and recommendations for Further Research. *Journal of Neurotherapy, 12*(1), 5-43.

Sokhadze, E. M., Stewart, C., Hollifield, M., & Tasman, A. (2008). Event-related potential study of executive dysfunctions in a speeded reaction task in cocaine addiction. *Journal of Neurotherapy, 12*(14), 185-204.

Sokhadze, E. M., Singh, S., Stewart, C., Hollifield, M., El-Baz, A., & Tasman, A. (2008). Attentional bias to drug and stress-related potential study of executive dysfunctions in a speeded reaction task in cocaine addiction comorbid with posttraumatic stress disorder. *Journal of Neurotherapy, 12*(4), 205-225.

Sokhadze, E. M., Stewart, C. M., & Hollifield, M. (2007). Integrating cognitive neuroscience research and cognitive behavioral treatment with neurofeedback therapy in drug addiction comorbid post-traumatic stress disorder: A conceptual review. *Journal of Neurotherapy, 11*(2), 13-44.

Solomon, A. (2001). *The noonday demon: An atlas of depression.* Memoir. New York, NY: Simon & Schuster.

Spiegelman, E. (2015). *Rewired: A bold new approach to addiction and recovery.* Hobart, NY: Hatherleigh Press.

Spiegelman, E. (2018). *The Rewired life: Creating a better life through self-care and emotional awareness.* Hobart, NY: Hatherleigh Press.

St. Clair, M. (2008). LENS Case Study: Traumatic brain injury from AVM (arterial venous malformation). *Neuroconnections, 7*(29-30).

Stange, J. P., Jenkins, L. M., Pocius, S., et al. (2019, October 10). Using resting-state intrinsic network connectivity to identify suicide risk in mood disorders. *Psychological Medicine, 10*, 1-11. doi:10.1017/S0033291719002356

Stevens, J. (1994). *Transforming your dragons: Turning personality fear patterns into personal power.* Santa Fe, NM: Bear & Co.

Stein, J. B., & Wargo, E. M. (2018). New reasons counselors should address smoking in their patients. *Advances in Addiction Recovery* (Fall), pp. 22-23.

Stein, M. B., & Walker, J. R. (2009). *Triumph over shyness: Conquering social anxiety disorder.* Silver Spring, MD: Anxiety Disorders Association of America.

Stitt, B. R. (2003). *Food and Behavior: A Natural Connection.* Manitowoc, WI: Natural Press. Anxiety Disorders Association of America (ADAA).

Stoller, C. C., Gruel, J. H., Cimmi, L. S., Fowler, M. S., Koonar, J. A. (2012). Effects of sensory-enhanced yoga on symptoms of combat stress in deployed military personnel. *American Journal of Occupational Therapy, 1*(66), 59-68.

Stoller, D. R., & Hill, B. A. (2013). *Coping with concussion and mild traumatic brain injury.* New York, NY: Penguin Random House.

Stowell, K., & Gary, S. (2004). *Understanding the addicted brain: From science to science.* Providence, RI: Manisses Communications Group, Inc.

Sullivan, E. V., & Pfefferbaum, A. (2009). Neuroimaging of the Wernicke-Korsakoff syndrome. *Alcohol and Alcoholism, 44*(2), 155-165.

Subramaniam, G. A., & Volkow, N. D. (2014). Substance misuse among adolescents: to screen or not to screen? *JAMA Pediatrics, 168*(9), 798-799. http://www.ncbi.nlm.nih.gov/pmc/articles/PMC4827336/

Sullivan M. A., Bisaga, A., Mariani, J. J., et al. (2013). Naltrexone treatment for opioid dependence: does its effectiveness depend on testing the blockade? *Drug Alcohol Dependence, 133*, 80-85.

Szalavitz, M. (2017). *Unbroken brain: A revolutionary new way of understanding addiction*. London, UK: Picador.

Sweeton, J. (2019). *Trauma treatment toolbox: 165 brain-changing tips, tools & handouts to move therapy forward*. Eau Claire, WI: PESI Publishing.

Tam, J. K., Warne, K. E., Meza, E. R. (2016). Smoking and the reduced life expectancy of individuals with serious mental illness. *American Journal of Preventive Medicine, 51*(6), 958–966.

Tan, G., Dao, T. K., Smith, D. L., Robinson, A., & Jensen, M. P. (2010). Incorporating complementary and alternative medicine (CAM) therapies to expand psychological services to veterans suffering from chronic pain. *Psychological Services, 7*(3), 148-161.

Tanielian, T. L., & Jaycox, L. H. (2008). *Invisible wounds of war: Psychological and cognitive injuries*. Santa Monica, CA: Rand.

Taub, E., & Rosenfeld, J. P. (1994). Is alpha-theta training the effective component of the alpha-theta therapy package for the treatment of alcoholism? *Biofeedback, 22*(3), 12-14.

Taxman, F. S., Perdoni, M. K., & Harrison, L. D. (2007). Drug treatment services for adult offenders. *Journal of Substance Abuse Treatment, 32*(3), 239–254.

Teetotaler, I. (2007). *Known cures for alcoholism & other drug addictions*. (Recovery journal). (n.p.): Day By Day recovery Resources.

Thatcher, R. W. (2000). EEG operant conditioning (biofeedback) and traumatic brain injury. *Clinical Electroencephalography, 31*, 38-44.

Thaut, M. H., & McIntosh, G. C. (2010). *How music helps to heal the injured brain: Therapeutic use crescendos thanks to advances in brain science*. Cerebrum. Retreived from https://www.dcconferences.com.au/wcnr2012/pdf/Cerebrum_Thaut_2010.pdf

Thompson, A. D., Guerrini, I., & Marshall, E. J. (2012). The evolution and treatment of Korsakoff's syndrome: Out of sight, out of mind? *Neuropsychology Review. 22*(2), 81-92.

The New Medicine. (2005). *About integrative medicine | Molecules of emotion*. Twin Cities Public Television. http://www.thenewmedicine.org/timeline/molecules_of_emotion.html

Theunissen, E. L., Hutten, N., Mason, N. L., Toennes, S. W., Kuypers, K. P. C., & Ramaekers, J. G. (2019, March 13). Neurocognition and subjective experience following acute doses of the synthetic cannabinoid JWH-018: Responders versus nonresponders. *Cannabis and Cannabinoid Research, 4*(1). https://doi.org/10.1089/can.2018.0047

Thomas, J. E., & Sattlberger, B. A. (1997). Treatment of chronic anxiety disorder with neurotherapy: A case study. *Journal of Neurotherapy 2*(2), 14-19.

Thomas, P., & Margulis, J. (2018). *The addiction spectrum: A compassionate. Holistic approach to recovery.* Harper Collins, New York, NY.

Thornton, K. (2000). Improvement/rehabilitation of memory functioning with neurotherapy/QEEG biofeedback. *Journal of Head Trauma Rehabilitation, 15*(6), 1285-1296.

Thornton, K., & Carmody, D. P. (2005). Electroencephalogram biofeedback for reading disability and traumatic brain injury. *Child & Adolescent Psychiatric Clinics of North America, 14*(1), 137-162.

Thornton, K., & Carmody, D. P. (2008). Efficacy if traumatic brain injury rehabilitation: interventions of QEEG-guided biofeedback, computers, strategies and medications. *Applied Psychophysiology & Biofeedback, 33,* 101-124.

Tilghman, A., & McGarry, B. (2013, March). Medicating the military: Use of psychiatric medication has spiked; concerns surface about suicide, other dangers. *Military Times.* Available from https://www.militarytimes.com/2013/03/29/medicating-the-military-use-of-psychiatric-drugs-has-spiked-concerns-surface-about-suicide-other-dangers/

Tinius, T. P., & Tinius, K. A. (2001). Changes after EEG biofeedback and cognitive retraining in adults with mild traumatic brain injury and attention deficit disorder. *Journal of Neurotherapy, 4*(2), 27-44.

Trammell, P. (2017). *Alcoholics not anonymous, a modern way to quit drinking.* Self Published.

Tremlow, S. W., & Bowen, W. T. (1976). EEG biofeedback induced self-actualization in alcoholics. *Journal of Biofeedback, 3,* 20-25.

Tremlow, S. W., & Bowen, W. T. (1977). Sociocultural predictors of self-actualization in EEG biofeedback treated alcoholics. *Psychological Reports, 40,* 591-598.

Tremlow, S. W., Sizemore, D. G., & Bowen, W. T. (1977). Biofeedback induced energy redistribution in the alcoholic EEG. *Journal of Biofeedback, 3,* 14-19.

Trevisan, L. A., Boutros, N., Ismene, M. D., Petrakis, L., & Krystal, J. H. (1998). Complications of alcohol withdrawal: pathophysiological insights. *Alcohol Health & Research World, 22*(1), 61-66.

Triffleman, E., Carroll, K., & Kellogg, S. (1999). Substance dependence posttraumatic stress disorder therapy: An integrated cognitive-behavioral approach. *Journal of Substance Abuse Treatment, 17*(1), 3-14.

Trudeau, D. L. (2000). A review of the treatment of addictive disorders by EEG biofeedback. *Clinical Electroencephalography, 31*, 14-26.

Trudeau, D. L. (2000). The treatment of addictive disorders by brain wave biofeedback: A review in suggestions for future research. *Clinical Electroencephalography, 31*(1), 13-22.

Trudeau, D. L. (2005). Applicability of brain wave biofeedback too substance use disorder in adolescents. *Child and Adolescent Clinics of North America, 14*, 125-136.

Trudeau, D. L. (2005). EEG biofeedback for addictive disorders – The state of the art in 2004. *Journal of Adult Development, 12*, 139-146.

Trudeau, D. L. (2008). Brainwave biofeedback for addictive disorder. *Journal of Neurotherapy, 12*(4), 181-183.

Trudeau, D. L. (2017). Experiences with alpha/theta: Its origins in studies of meditation. In A. Martins-Mourao & C. Kerson (Eds.), Alpha-theta neurofeedback in the 21st century A handbook for clinicians and researchers. *Neurofeedback and Neuromodulation Research*, Murfreesboro, TN. pp. 75-106.

Trudeau, D. L., Anderson, J., Hansen, L. M., Shagalov, D. N., Schmoller, J., Nugent, S., & Barton, S. (1998). Findings of mild traumatic brain injury in combat veterans with PTSD and a history of blast concussion. *The Journal of Neuropsychiatry and Clinical Neurosciences* (Summer), *10*(3), 308-13.

Trudeau, D. L., Sokhadze, T. M., & Cannon, R. L. (2009). Neurofeedback in alcohol and drug dependency. In T. H. Budzynski, H. K. Budzynski, J. R. Evans & A. Abarbanel (Eds.), *Introduction to quantitative EEG and neurofeedback: Advanced theory and applications*, pp. 241-268, Academic Press, Amsterdam.

Trudeau, D. L., Thuras, P., & Stockley, H. (1999). Quantitative EEG findings associated with chronic stimulant and cannabis abuse an ADHD in an adult male substance use disorder population. *Clinical Electroencephalography, 30*, 165-174.

Tumolo, J. (2019, September 18). *Meta-Review finds support for Omega-3 as adjunctive depression treatment*. Psychiatry and Behavioral Health Learning Network. Retrieved from www.psychcongress.com

Tumolo, J. (2019, October 23). *Brain scans differ in people with history of suicide attempt*. Psychiatry and Behavioral Health Learning Network. Retrieved from www.psychcongress.com

Tysvaer, A. T., Stroll, O. V., & Bachen, I. (1998). Soccer injuries to the brain: A neurologic and electroencephalographic study of former players. *Acta Neurologica Scandanavia, 80*, 151-156.

Uhl, G., Blum, K., Noble, E., & Smith, S. (1993). Substance abuse vulnerability and D2 receptor genes. *Trends in Neuroscience, 16*, 83-88.

US Department of Health and Human Services (HHS), Office of Attorney General (2016). Chapter 2. *The neurobiology of substance use, misuse, and addiction*. In (Ed.), Facing Addiction in America: The Surgeon General's Report on alcohol, drugs and health. Washington, DC. Available from https://addiction.surgeongeneral.gov/

US Department of Health and Human Services (HHS), Office of Attorney General (2016). Chapter 5. *Recovery: The many paths to wellness*. In (Ed.), Facing Addiction in America: The Surgeon General's Report on alcohol, drugs and health. Washington, DC. Available from https://addiction.surgeongeneral.gov/

US Department of Health and Human Services (HHS), Office of Attorney General (2016). Chapter 3. *Prevention programs and policies*. In (Ed.), Facing Addiction in America: The Surgeon General's Report on alcohol, drugs and health. Washington, DC. Available from https://addiction.surgeongeneral.gov/

US Department of Veteran Affairs. (2012). National Center for PTSD. http://www.ptsd.va.gov/

van der Hart, O., van Dijke, A., van Son, M., & Steele, K. (2002). Somatoform dissociation in traumatized World War I combat soldiers: A neglected clinical heritage. *Journal of Trauma and Dissociation, 7*(4), 33-66.

van der Kolk, B. A. (1994). The body keeps score: Memory and the evolving psychobiology of post-traumatic stress. *Harvard Review of Psychiatry, 1*(5), 253-265.

van der Kolk, B. A. (2004). Psychobiology of posttraumatic stress disorder. In J. Pankdeep (Ed.). *Biological Psychiatry*, (pp. 319-344). Wiley Liss, Hoboken, NJ.

van der Kolk, B. A. (2006). Clinical implications of neuroscience research in PTSD. *Annals of New York Academy of Sciences, 1077*(2), 77-293. https://doi.org/10.1196/annals.1364.022

van der Kolk, B. A. (2014). *The body keeps score: Brain, mind and body in the healing of trauma*. New York, NY: Viking.

van der Kolk, B. A., Hodgdon, H., Gapen, M., Musicaro, R., Savak, M. K., Hamlin, E., & Spinazzola, J. (2016). A randomized controlled study of neurofeedback for chronic PTSD. *PloS One, 11*(12), eo166752. https://doi.org/10.1371/journal.pone.0166751

VanHouten, J., et al. (2019 January 11). Drug overdose deaths among women aged 30–64 years — United States, 1999–2017. *Morbidity and Mortality Weekly Report, 68*, 1. doi:10.15585/mmwr.mm6801a1

Vernon, D., Frick, A., & Gruzelier, J. (2004). Neurofeedback a treatment for ADHD: A methodological review with implications for future research. *Journal of Neurotherapy, 8*(2), 53-82.

Veselak, C. (2020). *The Pro-Recovery Diet: The second essential factor in successful addiction recovery.* Alliance For Addiction Solutions. Available from https://www.allianceforaddictionsolutions.com/single-post/2020/01/21/The-Pro-Recovery-Diet-a-Successful-Addiction-Recovery-Meal-Plan

Volkow, N. D. (1995). Is Methylphenidate (Ritalin) like cocaine? *Archives of General Psychiatry, 52,* 456-463.

Volkow, N. D. (2003). Profile. National Institute on Drug Abuse. http://www.drugabuse.gov/about-nida/directors-page.html.

Volkow, N. D. (2004). *The neurobiology of drug abuse. In K. Stovell & S. Gray (Eds.), Understanding the addicted brain: From science to science.* Providence, RI: Manisses Communications Group, Inc.

Volkow, N. D. (2006, August 19). Treat the addict, cut the crime rate. *The Washington Post,* 66.

Volkow, N. D., Fowler, S. J., Wang, G. J., et al. (1999). Association of methylphenidate-induced craving with changes in right striato-orbitofrontal metabolism in cocaine abusers: Implications in addiction. *American Journal of Psychiatry, 156*(1), 19-26.

Volkow, N. D., Fowler, J. S., & Wang, G. J. (2003). The addicted human brain: Insights from imaging studies. *Journal of Clinical Investigation, 111*(10), 444-451.

Volkow, N. D., Fowler, J. S., & Wang, G. J. (2004). The addicted human brain viewed in light of imaging studies Brain circuits and treatment strategies. *Neuropharmacology, 47,* 3-13.

Volkow, N. D., & Li, T. K. (2005). Drugs and alcohol: Treating and preventing abuse, addiction and their medical consequences. *Pharma & Therapeutics, 108,* 3-17.

Volkow, N. D., Wang, G. J., Telang, F., et al. (2006). Cocaine cues and dopamine in dorsal striatum: mechanism of craving in cocaine addiction. *Journal of Neuroscience, 26,* 6583-6588.

Volkow, N. D., & McLellan, A. (2011). Curtailing diversion and abuse of opioid analgesics without curtailing pain treatment. *JAMA, 305*(13), 1346-1347.

Volkow, N. D., McLellan, T. A., Cotto, J. H., Karithanom, M. & Weiss, S. R. B. (2011). Characteristics of opioid prescriptions in (2009). *JAMA, 305*(13), 299–1301.

Volkow, N. D., Tomasi, D., Wang, G. J., et al. (2014). Stimulant-induced dopamine increases are markedly blunted in active cocaine abusers. *Mol Psychiatry, 19,* 1037-1043.

Volkow, N. D., & Koob, G. F. (2015). Brain disease model of addiction: why is it so controversial? *Lancet Psychiatry, 2*, 677-679.

Volkow, N. D., & Morales, M. (2015). The brain on drugs: from reward to addiction. *Cell, 162*, 712-725.

Volkow, N. D., Kobb, G. F., & McClellan, A. T. (2016). Neurobiologic advances from the brain disease model of addiction. *N England J Med, 374*, 363-371. doi:10.1056/NEJMra1511480

Walker, J. (2004). A neurologist's advice for mental health professionals o the use of QEEG and neurofeedback. *Journal of Neurotherapy, 8*(2), 97-100.

Walker, J. E. (2013). QEEG neurofeedback for anger/anger control disorder. *Journal of Neurotherapy, 17*(1). http://dx.doi.org/10.1080/10874208.2012.705767

Walker, J. E., & Lawson, R. (2013). Beta training for drug-resistant depression: A new protocol that usually reduces depression and keeps it reduced. *Journal of Neurotherapy, 17*(3). http://dx.doi.org/10.1080/10874208.2013.785784

Walters, D. (1998). EEG neurofeedback for alcoholism. *Biofeedback, 26*, 18-21.

Walwyn, W. M., Miotto, K. A., & Evans, C. J. (2010). Opioid pharmaceuticals and addiction: The issues, and research directions seeking solutions. *Drug and Alcohol Dependence, 108*(3), 156-165.

Wanberg, K. W., & Milkman, H. B. (1998). *Criminal conduct and substance abuse treatment: Strategies for self-improvement and change.* Thousand Oaks, CA: Sage.

Wang, S. Y. (2010). *The neuroscience of everyday life.* Chantilly, VA: Great Courses.

Wang, S. Y. (2012). New view of depression: An ailment of the entire body. *The Wall Street Journal.* Available from https://www.wsj.com/articles/SB10001424052702 3045877045773333941351135910

Wang, S. Y., Lin, I. M., Peper, E., Chen, Y. T., Tang, T. C., Yeh, Y. C., & Chu, C. C. (2016). The efficacy of neurofeedback among patients with major depressive disorder: Preliminary study. *NeuroRegulation, 3*(3), 127–134. Available from http://www.neuroregulation.org/article/view/16388

Warner, J. (2009). Can a veteran's court help former GIs find justice here at home? *Westword.* Available from https://www.westword.com/news/can-a-veterans-court-help-former-gis-find-justice-here-at-home-5107012

Watson, C. G., Herder, J., & Passini, F. T. (1978). Alpha biofeedback therapy in alcoholics: An 18-month follow-up. *J of Clinical Psychology, 34*(2), 765-769.

Weinberger, A. H, Platt, J., Esan, H., Galea, S., Erlich, D., & Goodwin, R. D. (2017). Cigarette smoking is associated with increased risk of substance use disorder relapse: a nationally representative, prospective longitudinal investigation. *The Journal of Clinical Psychiatry, 2*(78), e152-e160.

Webster, M. (2005). Predicting aberrant behaviors in opioid-treated patient: Preliminary validation of the opioid risk tool. *Pain Medicine, 6*(6), 432-442.

Weinhold, J. B., & Weinhold, B. K. (2011). *Healing developmental trauma: A systems approach to counseling individuals, couples, & families.* Denver, CO: Love Pub.

Weinhold, B. K. (2015). *Breaking free: Identifying and changing our addictive family patterns.* Colorado Springs, CO: CIRCL Press.

Weinhold, B. K., & Weinhold, J. B. (2015). *Developmental trauma: The game changer in the mental health profession.* Colorado Springs, CO: CIRCL Press.

Weil, A. (1995). *Spontaneous healing: How to discover and enhance your body's natural ability to maintain and heal itself.* New York, NY: Ballantine Books.

Westra, H. A., & Stewart, S. H. (1998). Cognitive behavioral therapy and pharmacotherapy: Complementary or contradictory approaches to the treatment of anxiety? *Clinical Psychology Review, 18*(3), 307-340.

White Bison. (2002). *The red road to wellbriety: The Native American ways.* Colorado Springs, CO: White Bison, Inc.

White, C. (2008, April). Letter to the editor: Restoring optimal brain function helps many health problems. Townsend Letter, *The Examiner of Alternative Medicine.* Available from http://www.townsendletter.com/April2008/ltr_white0408.htm

White, N. E., & Richards, L. (2009). Alpha-theta neurotherapy and the neurobehavior treatment of addictions, mood disorders and trauma. In T. H. Budzynski, H. K. Budzynski, J. R. Evans & A. Abarbanel (Eds.), *Introduction to Quantitative EEG and Neurofeedback: Advanced Theory and Applications* (2nd Edition). Academic Press, Amsterdam.

Whitney, D. (2020, January). Saving your loved ones from addiction by treating the disease in the brain and restoring hope. *The Sober World.* Available from https://www.thesoberworld.com/2020/01/01/saving-your-loved-ones-from-addiction-by-treating-the-disease-in-the-brain-and-restoring-hope/

Wigton, N. L. (2015). A review of QEEG-guided neurofeedback. *NeuroRegulation, 2*(3).

Wilford, B. B., & Dupont, R. L. (2007). Prescription drug abuse. In A. Wertheimer & T. Fields (Eds.), *A Textbook Pharmaceutical Policy.* Binghamton, NY: Haworth Press.

Williams, J. M., & Ziedonis, D. (2004). Addressing tobacco among individuals with a mental illness or an addiction. *Addictive Behaviors, 29*(6), 1067–1083.

Wilson, B. A. (1990). Cognitive rehabilitation for brain injured adults. In D. B. G., R. J. Sean, & A. H. Van Zomeren (Eds.), *Traumatic Brain Injury: Clinical Social and Rehabilitation Aspects.* Amsterdam: Swets & Zeitlinger, Pub. pp. 121-143.

Wilson, J. P. (1989). Trauma, transformation, and healing: An integrative approach to theory, research, and posttraumatic theory. New York, NY: Burnner/Mazel.

Wing, K. (2001). Effect of neurofeedback on motor recovery of a patient with brain injury: A case study and its implication for stroke rehabilitation. *Topics in Stroke Rehabilitation, 8*(3), 45-50.

Wood, J. (2019). For some, hyperactive neurons may hinder antidepressant effects. *Psych Central.* Available from https://psychcentral.com/news/2019/02/02/for-some-hyperactive-neurons-may-hinder-antidepressant-effects/142564.html

World of Molecules. (2012). Molecules of Emotion. http://www.worldofmolecules.com/emotions/

World Population Review. (2019, October 24). *Incarceration rates by country population.* Retrieved from http://worldpopulationreview.com/countries/incarceration-rates-by-country/

Wright, J. (2013). When Johnny comes marching home, again…he goes to jail. Available from http://www.ejfi.org/Courts/Courts-37.htm.

Wutke, M. (1992). Addiction, awakening and EEG biofeedback. *Biofeedback, 20*(2), 8-22.

Yalom, I. D., & Leszch, M. (2005). *The theory and practice of group psychotherapy* (5th ed.). New York: Basic Books. p. 272.

Yucha, C., & Gilbert, C. (2008). Evidence-based practice in biofeedback and neurofeedback. *Applied Psychophysiology and Biofeedback*, Wheatridge, CO. Available from https://www.aapb.org/files/public/Yucha-Gilbert_EvidenceBased2004.pdf

Zorumski, C. F. (2019, October 2). An update on GABA for clinicians. Presented at the Psych Congress 2019, *Practical Psychopharmacology* Pre-Conference: San Diego, CA.

www.ingramcontent.com/pod-product-compliance
Lightning Source LLC
Chambersburg PA
CBHW060844280326
41934CB00007B/909